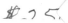

The Complete Guide To A Fast Keto Diet For Beginners

Ketogenic Diet Recipes And Meal Plans For People On The Go

Hub Spoke Publishing

Suzanne Summers

Table Of Contents

Introduction 1

CHAPTER 1 What Is Keto, Ketogenic? 4

CHAPTER 2 Let's Chat About Ketosis 6

CHAPTER 3 So….What Should We Do Next? 13

CHAPTER 4 All Planned Out And Ready! 26

CHAPTER 5 Oh Something's Cookin 46

CHAPTER 6 Questions You Will Ask 152

CONCLUSION 154

Resources 155

This Page Intentionally Left Blank

Introduction

A Little Bit About Me

As I sit here typing this book I am flooded with memories of my life before the ketogenic diet. I was stuck in a body I wasn't happy with and a way of eating that made me feel anything but good about myself. After years of yo-yo dieting and losing and regaining the same 20 pounds, I knew it was time for a change.

Now, as you are probably aware, there is literally an ocean of diet plans out there to choose from. I had already done a bunch, including fad diets that didn't really work in the long-term. So, how do you know which one to choose?

Well, for starters, you must change your thought process. You see, for so many years I was looking for the perfect diet. Guess what? It doesn't exist. I've learned over the years that diets are temporary fixes that typically cannot be sustained over the long haul. I needed to find a way of eating that I could commit to for the rest of my life.

Thus, began my search. I read books, visited Facebook groups, watched documentaries, and even visited a nutritionist. My mind was flooded with words like, "low-fat", "calorie restriction", and "low-carb". I literally had to take a seat in my office (which is actually a hike on a wooded bike trail) and think about all the information I received.

There was one way of eating (WOE) that I kept coming back to. During my research, I continually saw the word "keto". At the time, I had no clue as to what that even was. After determining that it was some sort of low-carb diet, I chalked keto up to be an Atkins plan.

Boy, was I ever wrong!

After returning from my hike, I went into my actual office, sat down at the computer, and started to research this keto thing a bit more.

Ladies and gentlemen, the scales had been removed from my eyes.

Keto, or rather the ketogenic diet, is not an Atkins Plan at all. Yes, there are similarities, but keto is focused on eating high healthy fats and moderate protein. The Atkins plan is the opposite. However, each WOE focuses on very low-carb.

What caught my eye about the keto WOE is that you got to eat FAT. Have you ever heard of such a thing? Eating fat to lose weight? I had always been taught that fat makes you fat. That is so not true, and I'll cover why as you dive deeper into this book.

I knew, from that point on, that I wanted to give keto a try. You get to eat fatty foods like burgers, bacon, and butter. Who wouldn't want to do that? Plus, you lose weight in the process.

I totally immersed myself in the science behind this WOE and was impressed by what I found. I was glad to know that the ketogenic diet was not a fad diet or trend. This WOE has strong roots and has been around since the 1920s.

Over the course of a year, I stayed true to keto and the results were more than I ever could have imagined. Not only did I lose weight, but I felt better and certain health issues in my life improved.

We've all been in a place where we needed something special in our lives to really take hold of who we are and change us for the better. Keto did that for me. I was sick and tired of being sick and tired. For me, the key to a drastic change was within the foods I was eating. This is the case with most people.

I want you to know that I've been overweight, and I haven't liked who I saw in the mirror, just like you. I know what it feels like to go to the store and leave in tears because the clothes just don't fit right.

I also know what it feels like to be successful in an eating plan.

The days of losing and regaining the same weight are over for me and they can be for you, too. Keto changed my entire world and how I think about food and dieting.

I am not a doctor or a dietician but rather a woman who got tired of yo-yo dieting and wanted a new lease on life. It is my intention that this book will open your eyes to the wonderful world of keto, that has been backed by science, and change your life like it changed mine.

Who This Book Is For

Essentially, this book is for everyone. Keto focuses on zapping the sugar out of your life and there isn't one person on this planet whose health didn't improve from doing that. However, there are some specific folks out there that keto is targeted towards.

Here's a list of questions to ask yourself:

- Do I want to lose weight?
- Do I want to maintain my weight after I have lost it?
- Do I have health issues that need to be reversed?
- Do I desire to eat a healthier diet?
- Do I want to feel energized throughout my entire day?

If you answered "yes" to at least one of these questions this book is probably for you. Keto is designed with all types in mind. It is a WOE that can help anyone, and everyone feel better, look better, and even think better.

What This Book Provides

In addition to a wealth of information, this book gives you easy-to-understand meal plans that are well thought out, tasty, and perfect for your busy lifestyle. I not only include 1 meal plan, but 2. The second plan focuses on simple meals that can be prepped and prepared quickly. So, even if you are a busy mom, a working dad, or a young student at college, you can still create keto meals that are tailored towards your on-the-go lifestyle.

Don't worry. These meal plans come with step-by-step recipes, ingredient lists, and even nutritional information. I've literally done all the legwork for you. All you have to do is turn the pages of this book.

This book also contains a detailed section on how to get started with the ketogenic lifestyle. There is a little something called "ketosis" and I'll give you the tools to help you better understand what that is and how to get your body into it.

What's a weight-loss and healthy eating book without the bones to back it up? Not very good. That's why I've included scientific evidence throughout this entire book, so you know what you're reading is legit and not just a bunch of hogwash. By the time you finish reading you'll have an in-depth understanding of the ketogenic diet and why it works.

Lastly, I provide you with strategies and tips to make keto work for you forever. If you're anything like me, you are tired of diets that don't work. You'll learn how to sustain your new keto lifestyle without getting burnt out in the process.

So, are you ready to get started on your keto journey? Yes? Great! Let's do it!

CHAPTER 1
What Is Keto, Ketogenic?

<u>What is the Ketogenic Diet?</u>

To simply put it, the ketogenic diet (keto) is a high healthy fat, moderate protein, and very low-carb way of eating (WOE). Many folks confuse keto with the Atkin's Plan, and although there are similarities, Atkins focuses on high protein, moderate fat, and low-carb intake. In the big scheme of things, these are major differences.

So, you may be wondering, "Why choose keto"? Well, my friend, there are many reasons as to why the keto WOE might be good for you. For starters, the keto diet is backed by evidential science. There have been over <u>20 studies</u> showing the efficacy of a high-fat, low-carb (HFLC) diet that helps people lose weight and improve health (<u>1</u>).

The keto WOE is so much more than just a weightless plan. There are studies that have proven it to combat diabetes, cancer, seizure disorders, and even Alzheimer's Disease (<u>2</u>, <u>3</u>, <u>4</u>, <u>5</u>).

Moving on...

So, what happens when you drastically reduce your carbohydrate intake and increase the amount of healthy fats that you eat? Your body goes into a metabolic state called ketosis. Ketosis involves the body producing ketones and using them for energy instead of sugar (carbs).

Ketosis is something that you want to have happen. Depending on your body, it can take anywhere from a few hours to a few days to reach a state of ketosis. Once you jumped over into ketosis territory, your body will begin the process of learning how to burn fat for energy once all the ketones have been used up. In addition, the fat in your liver will turn into ketones and these ketones can supply energy for your brain. Say goodbye to brain fog, people (<u>6</u>, <u>7</u>)!

Many people who struggle with blood sugar problems such as diabetes and insulin resistance have noticed an extreme decrease in blood glucose levels. There are many benefits to having your blood sugar balanced (<u>8</u>).

<u>Summary</u>

The ketogenic diet is a healthy high fat, moderate protein, very low-carbohydrate WOE that balances blood sugars and naturally shifts the body's metabolism away from carbohydrates and plunges it into the land of ketones and fat.

Exploring the different Types of Ketogenic WOE's

You probably didn't know this but there are a few different ways to approach the ketogenic diet. Let's take a look at them:

- Standard Keto diet (SKD) – This is the type of keto WOE that most people start with as it is cut and dry and easy to follow and maintain. It is very high healthy fat, moderate in protein, and very low-carb. Normally, the diet follows a 75% fat, 20% protein, and 5% carbs ratio.
- Cyclical ketogenic diet (CKD): This WOE allows you to have times of higher carb eating. For example, you may have 5 very strict SKD days followed by 2 high-carbohydrate days. Some folks refer to this as "refeeding".
- Targeted ketogenic diet (TKD) – If you are an athlete or body builder, TKD may be the type of keto WOE that works best for you as it allows you to add carbs centered around your workouts.
- High-protein ketogenic diet – This type of keto WOE is pretty similar to a SKD, but it allows for more protein consumption. The ratio looks something like 60% fat, 35% protein, and 5% carbs.

Keep in mind, when choosing a ketogenic WOE, only the SKD and high-protein methods have been researched and studied extensively. The other keto diets mentioned are a bit more advanced and widely used in the athlete/body builder communities.

Overall, the SKD is the most researched and most recommended of the four.

At the end of the day, only you know the right ketogenic diet style to engage in. Perhaps, talking over the different styles with your doctor will be helpful, too. More than likely, unless you're an extreme athlete, the SKD will be your go-to.

CHAPTER 2
Let's Chat About Ketosis

Why is Being in Ketosis Important?

So, we touched briefly on ketosis in chapter 1 and now we will explore it a bit further. It's important that you have a good understanding of what ketosis is, how it works, and why you need your body to be in it while eating a ketogenic diet.

What is Ketosis?

As previously stated, ketosis is a metabolic state in which carbs no longer work as the main source of energy for the body. Instead, your body uses ketones and then fat for fuel.

When you stop feeding your body carbs (sugar) it has limited access to glucose, which it uses for fuel. You see, when there is glucose in your body you will always burn it first because when glucose levels become to high, it can be deadly. Your body is smart and knows just what to do to keep you alive. There are malfunctions in this process when someone is a diabetic.

Here's a fun fact. Babies are born in a state of ketosis. One might argue that being in ketosis is more natural than using carbs for fuel. I'd say that they are right since we come into the world this way (9). Ketosis also happens during pregnancy and when you are fasting.

In order to get yourself into a state of ketosis, you need to restrict your carbohydrate intake rather extremely. This means you should eat no more than 50 grams of carbs per day. Some folks need to keep their intake to around 20 grams of carbs while they ate first starting the keto diet.

You'll have to remove certain foods from your diet in order to make this happen. Toss out the candy, grains, sugar-laden soda pop, starchy vegetables, and fruit, to name a few.

As you decrease your carbohydrate intake, your insulin levels also decrease and fatty acids are released from your body fat reserves in quite hefty amounts.

Another interesting concept is that ketones can cross the blood-brain barrier and fatty acids cannot. Ketones give your brain a mega-boost of energy when glucose is not present. This is a very good thing.

Benefits of Being in Ketosis

Being in ketosis comes with many benefits and most of them are health and weight loss related. If you are dealing with certain health issues such as high blood pressure, diabetes, and fatty liver disease, being in ketosis can actually help reverse these ailments.

In addition to helping you combat serious health problems, being in ketosis can help you lose weight and maintain the loss. I don't know about you, but this aspect is one of my favorites parts of being in ketosis. Following a ketogenic diet can help you toss out those fat pants, forever.

Health

Diabetes – So, it is no wonder that following a ketogenic diet and being in a state of ketosis can help diabetics. The diet is all about restricting carbs (sugar) and nourishing the body with healthy fats. Since most diabetics practice carb restriction, anyway, the keto way of eating shouldn't be to hard for them. When these folks start adding healthy fats into the mix is when the magic happens.

Researchers conducted a 24-week study, in 2008, to understand and determine the effects of a low-carb diet on folks with type-2 diabetes (10). These people were also dealing with obesity. As the study concluded, subjects who followed the keto WOE saw marked improvements in their blood sugar levels and were even able to reduce their diabetes medication. The other test groups, who followed a low-glycemic diet, didn't have as good of results. Another study, performed in 2017, determined the ketogenic diet outshined a standard, low-fat diabetes diet over the course of 32 weeks in correlation to weight loss and A1c levels (11). Additionally, a 2013 review reports that the keto WOE can lead to impressive improvements in balancing blood glucose, lowering and stabilizing A1c levels, weight loss, and even help people get off their diabetes management medications more than any other diet (12).

Metabolic Syndrome – A very tough illness to beat, the signs of this syndrome include having a large midsection, high blood pressure, high triglyceride levels, low HDL levels, and high glucose levels. Unfortunately, this syndrome is linked with type 2 diabetes and cardiovascular disease.

Researchers at Bethel University of Minnesota conducted a study of three groups composed of adults with metabolic syndrome. One group followed the keto diet without exercise, the second ate a Standard American Diet (SAD) without exercise, and the third group followed a SAD diet with 30 minutes od exercise most days of the week.

The study concluded that the folks following the ketogenic diet with exercise had much more success than the other 2 groups did in terms of achieving weight loss and more effective against a large range of health disorders (13).

Brain issues – A common myth is that the brain needs 130 grams of carbohydrates to function. A report by the US Institute of Medicine's Food and Nutrition Board clearly debunks this myth and states that the brain can actually function on zero carbs (14).

Eating a ketogenic diet supply's energy for the brain by way of ketogenesis and gluconeogenesis (15).

One major issue of the brain is epilepsy and keto has shown to be a key component in easing the symptoms of this debilitating disorder. In fact, in 1924, the Classic Ketogenic Diet was created by doctors to help children suffering from epileptic seizures ([16]). This WOE is still used today to treat seizure disorders.

Cancer – Eating a ketogenic diet is known to weaken cancer cells. Studies have shown that sugar feeds cancer and creates an acidic environment within the body. When you consume a high-fat/low-carb diet you are essentially not giving cancer cells what they need to thrive. What happens? They die ([17])!

Reduces inflammation – When your body is inflamed you can experience all sorts of things such as arthritic pain and autoimmune issues. Eating excess sugar produces high amounts of insulin within your body which raises inflammatory markers and triggers chronic disease, Nixing the sugar and following a keto WOE can reverse these problems and help you to feel better ([18]).

Cholesterol – So, you've probably been taught that fat makes you fat and causes heart disease and high cholesterol, right? Well, research has proven this to be a myth. In fact, research has shown that sugar(carbs) make you fat and cause health issues like high triglyceride levels. Now, if you combine both carbs and fat together in your diet then yes, you are creating a recipe for disaster. Removing the carbs and enjoying healthy fats by themselves will do the opposite ([19]).

Blood Pressure – A study was conducted involving a few test groups who all had high blood pressure and were put on various diets like The Zone, Ornish, and Atkins. It was concluded that the Atkins group saw the highest decrease in both systolic and diastolic blood pressure ([20]). Granted, this study didn't include the keto diet, but it did prove that a low-carb diet is successful in lowering blood pressure.

Fatty Liver Disease – There are a number of factors that play into fatty liver disease. If you struggle from nonalcoholic fatty liver disease your lifestyle is the biggest culprit to why you have the disease in the first place. Eating much and exercising too little are key players in the game of fatty liver disease. Turning to a low-fat diet to correct fatty liver disease has been shown to be counterproductive and ineffective. However, keto has displayed some promising results ([21]).

Lifestyle

How will the ketogenic diet affect your life? Well, we've already established that if you are dealing with certain health ailments eating a ketogenic diet can help bring you relief. You'll also notice other areas of your life improving such as less fatigue, clearer thinking, more energy, and stabilized moods.

Sounds good to me!

Weight-loss – The ketogenic diet has been proven time and time again to help people lose weight. Removing carbs from the diet and being in a state of ketosis encourages your body to burn fat for fuel. When you use your fat stores for fuel you are losing fat on your body. This will cause the much-coveted weight-loss effect leaving you with a trimmer body and smaller clothes.

Hunger management/appetite control – When you begin increasing healthy fats into your diet you'll find yourself becoming satiated quicker and for longer periods of time. Fat tastes good and is very satisfying. Sugar (carbs) on the other hand, gives you a burst of energy and satisfies your hunger pains for a brief time but shortly, you'll notice you are craving sugar again and begin to feel sluggish. This is called a "sugar crash". It is important to understand that fat nourishes and satisfies your body while sugar inflames and increases your cravings.

Energy – As aforementioned, carbohydrates give you a temporary burst of fuel but that energy is quickly followed by a crash. When you are in ketosis and are being fueled by healthy fat, you'll experience sustained energy throughout your day.

Mental clarity – When your body starts using ketones for fuel and then fat, you'll notice that your brain fog will lift. You'll experience clearer thinking, better decision making, and an overall crisper thought process (22).

You'll burn fat for fuel – As we've been discussing this entire book so far, the keto WOE allows your body to burn fat for fuel and when you tell glucose to take a hike, well, all sorts of great things happen. You'll find yourself feeling better across the entire board.

Mood stabilization – When we aren't eating a healthy diet and consuming high amounts of sugar, we can become aggravated, moody, and overly emotional. Have you ever heard the term "hangry"? It means you are angry because you are hungry. Being "hangry" is due to your body craving carbohydrates. When on a ketogenic diet you won't be craving sugar and you'll feel more satiated which will ultimately lead to having better moods. The inflammation in your body will also improve which again, leads to the stabilization of your emotions.

<u>Is the Ketogenic Diet for You?</u>

Honestly, that is a question you need to ask yourself. Taking in all of the information that I've supplied you thus far, does it seem that keto would be a good fit for you? Do you have any health issues that might make keto difficult or unsafe?

I highly recommend that you speak with your family doctor before beginning the ketogenic WOE. In most cases, a doctor is going to give you his or her blessing to go forward with a low-carb diet. Why? Because most health care professionals aren't in the business of pushing high-sugar diets on their patients.

Please, understand, that I am not your doctor and the information in this book is not meant to treat or diagnose your health problems.

Whatever issues you may have going on with your health, please, talk them over with your doctor and tell him or her why you think a keto WOE is good for you. Glean your doctor's input.

Keto may not be appropriate for the following people who have the following health issues:

- Diabetes
- Kidney disease

- Liver or pancreatic disease
- Pregnant or nursing mothers
- People who actively have or are recovering from an eating disorder
- People recovering from surgery
- People who are underweight
- Children under the age of 18

If anything on the list above applies to you, please, understand that this doesn't mean you are automatically exempt from following a keto WOE. It just means you really need to talk your condition and keto over with your doctor before you begin. I highly recommend you follow the advice of your health care provider.

Ketoacidosis

You may have heard some hype between the ketogenic diet and ketoacidosis. I am here to explain the difference between the two because they are nothing alike, at all (23).

We've already been talking about what ketosis is so let's recap. Ketosis is the presence of ketones in the body and it is not harmful. You get into a state of ketosis by restricting carbohydrate intake.

Ketoacidosis (DKA) is an extremely serious condition that affects people who suffer from type 1 diabetes mellitus. It is a life-threatening condition and requires immediate medical help due to the presence of dangerously high amounts of ketones and blood sugar levels. When this happens, your blood becomes too acidic, which changes the way your bodily organs work.

There are a few things that can lead a person who suffers from type 1 diabetes mellitus into a state of ketoacidosis and they include illness, not eating properly, or not getting enough insulin. Very rarely is ketoacidosis brought on by eating a low-carb diet, especially in a person who is not diabetic.

Ketoacidosis can also develop in folks who suffer from type 2 diabetes who have very little to no insulin production.

Ketosis = Safe

Ketoacidosis = Very Dangerous

Again, I cannot stress this enough, if you suffer from underlying health problems, especially any form of diabetes, please talk over the ketogenic diet with your doctor before starting.

Ketoacidosis is very rare, even in people who are diabetic, and it is pretty much non-existent in a person who does not have diabetes.

Keto Flu

You may or may not have heard of the keto flu. There is a good possibility that you are reading this right now and thinking, "The flu?? Why on earth would I do a diet plan that gives me the flu?"

Woah, hold your horses, pardner! The keto flu is not the "flu" at all. There are no viruses or bacteria involved whatsoever. You don't need medication or a trip to the doctor. Actually, a few swigs of pickle juice will probably due the trick.

I'm sure I've just confused you even more. Pickle juice?

Okay, here's the 411 on the keto flu. When you restrict carbohydrates your body sort of goes into a panic. For years, you've lovingly fed your bed sugar and your body got used to that relationship. All of a sudden, you stop with the cookies, cakes, and breads and your body doesn't quite know how to handle the breakup.

This is when, a new follower of keto, you begin to feel a little bit terrible. However, don't worry, these flu-like symptoms are temporary and will subside once your body adjusts to eating a low-carb diet.

Symptoms of the Keto Flue include:

- Craving sugar
- Feeling dizzy
- Not being able to think clearly
- Grouchiness
- Lack of concentration/focus
- Upset stomach
- Feeling nauseous
- Muscle cramps
- Feeling confused
- Not being able to sleep

Now, you may or may not experience these symptoms. Some folks only experience a few while others experience them all. Keto flu truly depends on the individual and their personal metabolic flexibility. Metabolic flexibility is simply how well you can adapt to using a different energy source such as carbs, or fats. Your genetics and lifestyle deeply impact your metabolic flexibility.

As you restrict carbohydrates, water and sodium are flushed out of the body which can leave you a bit parched. Dehydration can make you feel those dreaded flu-like symptoms. A great rule of thumb is to always drink plenty of water while begging the ketogenic diet (you always should, anyway). What about that pickle juice? Pickle juice contains a ton of sodium which helps replenish those electrolytes. Taking a few sips can help you feel better.

Tips for remedying symptoms of the keto flu:

- Drinking water with a pinch of unrefined salt
- Supplement your diet with sodium, magnesium, and potassium
- Eat more fat
- Exercise – low-intensity
- Meditate
- Get adequate sleep

Things you should not do:

- High-intensity workouts
- Consume high amounts of protein
- Stress over uncontrollable things
- Eat carbs/sugar

So, remember, the keto flu is not dangerous, and it will most likely happen to you as you begin to cut carbs from your plate. Keep in mind that this is a transition that your body is going through and it to shall pass. Use the tips above to remedy your symptoms and keep on ketoing.

CHAPTER 3
So....What Should We Do Next?

Welcome to chapter 3! If you are still with me then it is clear you are serious about your keto journey. I'm proud of you.

So, we've learned a lot about the keto WOE up to this point and now it is time to jump into the fat of the diet (no pun intended). In this chapter you will learn how to get started in the ketogenic lifestyle. We'll cover all the basics that you need to know in order to be successful.

You might be feeling a little overwhelmed with all the information and new terms you are learning but don't worry. By the time you finish this chapter you are going to be ready to start keto like a champ.

Let's go!

KETO IN A NUTSHELL

Let's refresh a bit and go over the basic tenants of keto, shall we?

We know that the ketogenic diet is high in healthy fats, moderate in protein, and very low in carbohydrates.

We know that once you begin the ketogenic diet and restricting your carbs your body will fall into ketosis.

We know that ketosis is safe and not at all what ketoacidosis is. Ketosis means there are ketones in your blood and you are now burning them for fuel instead of glucose.

We know that you may or may not feel symptoms of the "keto flu" when you are still starting out.

We know not to worry about the keto flu because we understand how to combat it.

We know that the ketogenic WOE leads to sustainable weight-loss, better health, and more energy.

What else do we know?

Keto is amazing ☺

KNOW YOUR BODY

The very first stepping stone to starting a ketogenic diet is knowing your body. You need to know where you're at in terms of health, weight, and measurements. The best way to do this is to schedule a full-body exam with your doctor.

You'll want to go over any pre-existing health issues with your doctor and discuss how starting keto will impact them. If you learn you have other health problems, discuss those, too.

Ask your doctor to perform blood work on you. You'll want a full lipid panel profile at this starting point. It's great to know your numbers and then have them rechecked in 6 months or so and compare your progress.

You'll want to calculate your Body Mass Index (BMI). You can do this by dividing your weight in pounds by your height in inches. Then, divide your answer by your height again to get your individual BMI. You can also follow this same formula in kilograms and meters. To make things even easier, you can find a BMI calculator on-line and simply input your stats and let the robots do the figuring for you.

Make sure to weight yourself and record your answer so you can keep track of your progress.

You'll want to get measurements of your body. This is very important for those times when you don't see the scale moving as much as you'd like it to be. Many times, folks will see massive differences in inch-loss versus scale lose.

Measure your hips, calf, thigh, wrist, and forearm. You can do this by using a seamstress tape measure. Or, if you know of a local gym, perhaps a trainer there can do it for you. Make sure to record your findings so you can compare progress at a later time.

If you are on a budget and the thought of going to the doctor's office makes you cringe due to high medical costs, I've got some solutions for you.

Does your employer offer medical insurance or a health incentive plan? If you don't have access to health insurance, make sure to ask your doctor's finance department if they offer a discount for cash-paying patients. Most of the time, you'll be given as much as a 60% discount.

There are also programs you can sign up for that offer cost-sharing. This means that you pay a monthly fee of x amount of dollars as do other people from around the country. When you go to the doctor's office you submit your bills to the program and your fees are paid for.

If all else fails, you can easily weigh and measure yourself at home. You won't be able to perform a full-body exam or give yourself bloodwork but at least you'll know some starting point numbers.

I do recommend that you try your best to get in to see your health care professional at some point, though. You want to be sure all your parts are functioning properly, especially when starting a new diet plan.

WHAT IS YOUR "WHY"

This next section is very important, and it is something I really want you to think about. What is your "why'? Why are you deciding to start the keto WOE? What has motivated you to kick bad eating habits and get healthier?

Perhaps, you have health conditions that you want to improve, or you aren't at a weight that is acceptable to you. Maybe, you want to get healthier, so you can play with your children/grandchildren with ease and not always be sore and tired.

Whatever your "why" is, I want you to write it down and keep it some place handy so whenever you feel like giving up you can return to your "why" and remember what this is all for. When I started keto, I kept my "why" posted on the refrigerator so that I could see it every day. I've even heard of people keeping a sticky note on their bathroom mirror.

Another good thing you can do is journaling. Write out your thoughts as to why you are changing your lifestyle. Once you establish your "why" you can then start to list out some goals. Make sure your goals are realistic and attainable. You and I both know that making a goal to lose 50 pounds (unless you are morbidly obese) in a month is not realistic. However, 10 is.

I really want you to wrap your head around your "why" and give it some good thought. Your "why" will be your motivating factor to keep ketoing on.

If you aren't into writing things down, that's okay! As long as you can remember why you are doing this and it helps keep you disciplined, you're good. Maybe you can tattoo your "why' on your body? Just kidding ☺

KETONE MONITORING SUPPLIES: WHICH DO YOU USE?

Believe it or not, there are ways to know the level of ketones swirling around in your body. So folks in the ketogenic community are die-hard users of these devices while some think they are unnecessary. I fall somewhere in between. I feel that if you have these monitors, great, if you don't, also great.

Now, I will say, knowing that you are in ketosis when you first start the ketogenic diet is a plus. It is motivating and gives you the comfort that this keto thing is really working.

There are three types of monitors in which you can test yourself for the presence of ketones:

- Blood
- Breath
- Urine

Blood monitors are highly accurate but they are expensive. Plus, you must poke yourself in order to use them. Most folks don't relish the idea of playing in their own blood. Many people in the diabetic community opt for blood monitors because it gives them a concise estimate of their blood glucose and ketone levels. It also helps them keep an eye out for ketoacidosis.

Pros – Most accurate ketone testing method

Cons – Expensive and not very pleasant to use

Breath ketone monitors measure the amount of acetone in the breath. Yes, acetone as in the main ingredient in nail polish remover. Your breath may smell of this for a period of time as your body adjusts to the low-carb lifestyle. Measuring breath acetone can tell you whether you are in mild ketosis or not. This device is useful for people trying to establish a baseline of ketosis without needing to know how deeply they're into it.

Pro- - Easy to use and affordable

Cons – Isn't as in-depth as a blood monitor

Measuring ketones in your urine is extremely affordable an easy. You simply urinate into a cup and hold the dipstick in the urine for a few seconds. The more purple the color is the higher the concentration of ketones are in your body. Urine sticks, just like breath monitors, can determine whether you are in ketosis or not, but they cannot determine how deeply like blood monitoring can.

Pros – Easy to use and cheap

Cons – You need to collect urine. Not as effective as blood monitoring

So, in the end, unless you are a diabetic, I wouldn't spend the money on a blood monitoring system. If anything, the breath or urine ways of monitoring will work just fine. Many people, myself included, prefer breath monitoring because it is less messy than urine testing.

Please, remember, that if you can't afford these ketone testing supplies or you simply don't want them that that is perfectly fine. You really don't need them in order to be successful on the ketogenic diet as there are clear signs and symptoms of being ketosis as we discussed in chapter 2.

MACROS

You may or may not have heard of "macros" before which is short for macronutrients. Macronutrients are the energy-giving properties of the foods that we eat and they fuel our bodies. Macros consist of fat, protein, and carbohydrates. When embarking on a keto diet journey, knowing your personal macros is important because you need to have the right balance of fats, proteins, and carbs in order to get into ketosis and to stay there. You want your body to be a fat-burning powerhouse.

Let me further break macros down for you.

Carbohydrates are the only macronutrient that you do not need for survival. Fats and proteins are considered to be essential for survival, but carbs are not. For someone who is just getting started on the keto WOE you should aim for no more than 20 grams of carbohydrates per day.

Keep in mind, that carbs aren't just sugary cakes, cookies, and candy. Carbs are in vegetables, fruit, wheat, and bread. You must keep an eye on your intake of all carbs in all foods.

When you look at a food label you re going to see carbohydrates listed. You will also see fiber listed. What you want to do is find the NET CARB count. To do this, subtract the carbs from the fiber and that is the number you use. Fiber that occurs naturally in a food does not impact your glycemic index, so it basically cancels out some of the total carb count.

Protein is important in a ketogenic diet as it helps you preserve your lean body mass. The amount of protein you need will depend on the amount of lean body mass you already have. Check out these general guidelines for protein intake per the Ketogasm website (24):

- 0.7 to 0.8 grams of dietary protein per pound of muscle to preserve muscle mass
- 0.8 to 1.2 grams of dietary protein per pound of muscle to gain muscle mass

Keep in mind, you DO NOT want to lose muscle mass. You want to lose fat. I know many of you are just looking to lose weight no matter how it happens but losing muscle mass is not the way.

Getting adequate protein is important in the ketogenic diet, however, you don't want to go overboard with it as to much protein can be stressful to the kidneys.

Find your daily protein percentage by multiplying your body weight by your body fat percentage. Then subtract your body fat weight from your total weight and that will give you your lean body mass. Next, take your lean body mass amount and multiply it by your protein requirement ratio and you'll find the grams of protein you need on a daily basis to maintain your muscle mass.

Fat is an essential component to the ketogenic lifestyle. It is the macronutrient that satisfies your hunger pangs due to be so satiating. When wanting to maintain your weight you need to eat enough fat to support your total daily fuel expenditure. To lose weight, you'll need to eat a fat deficit.

Putting it All Together

So, the best way to find your personal macros is by using a macronutrient calculator. You can find one at the Ketogains website. These calculators make it super simple to find your individual macros. All you have to do is put your weight and body fat percentage in and the calculator will do the rest.

Your MACROS Will Change

As you begin to lose weight you will need to adjust your macros. I, personally, would make these adjustments every two weeks. It is so important to keep track of your weight, so you know how to figure your macronutrients. As your size begins to shrink so will your macros.

FOODS YOU SHOULD MAKE FRIENDS WITH

When it comes to keto, there are a few staple foods that you really should keep on hand just help yourself stay satiated and to encourage ketosis. The following list isn't a must-have, but it does help. I like to think of these foods as "keto staples".

- Coconut oil – This oil is super nourishing for the body. It is purely fat and great for helping you to get into ketosis. You also may want to consider using MCT (medium chain triglycerides) oil which is a concentrated form of coconut oil that is high in

Caproic, caprylic, capric, and lauric acids. These acids quickly turn into energy and metabolized in the body.

- Extra-virgin olive oil – Another oil that is high in healthy fat and great for using in homemade salad dressings and marinades. You don't want to use olive oil in high heat settings so save it for your favorite cold-recipes.
- Cheese – Cheese is probably one of my favorite keto-friendly foods. It's high in healthy fats, tastes wonderful, and very filling. You can use cheese in a variety of recipes. Feel free to consume any type of cheese you want including cream cheese. Keep in mind that processed cheese, like Velveeta, are not part of the keto equation as they contain sugar.
- Tree nut butter – Tree nut butters are an amazing source for both fat and protein. They taste great and are wonderful by the spoonful or in keto desserts. You can use peanut butter, but it needs to be a natural peanut butter without added sugar. When using any nut butters make sure to keep an eye on the ingredients and net carb count.
- Cauliflower – When it comes to keto veggies, cauliflower is the real deal. This powerhouse veggie is very low in carbs and can be used to create all sorts of substitutes like rice, noodles, and even pizza crust! There are tons of recipes that show you how to do this. You can even make faux mashed potatoes with cauliflower.
- Cod liver oil – Cod liver oil is chock full of omega 3's and is great for keeping your heart healthy. I wouldn't use this oil in recipes or for straight up eating as it tastes extremely fishy. However, finding yourself a good cod liver oil supplement is a wise move to make for the added cardiovascular benefits.
- Kelp – The best and easiest way to incorporate kelp into your diet is when it is in a powdered form. You may think it is super fishy tasting, but it really isn't! It's great for sprinkling on salads and even into keto-approved smoothies. I like to add kelp to tomato soup. Sea kelp is a natural source of vitamins A, B1, B2, C, D, and E and includes minerals zinc, iodine, magnesium, potassium, copper, and calcium.
- Avocado – If you choose to be on a ketogenic diet then you pretty much have to like avocados. Kidding! However, avocados are an excellent source of fat and they are quite versatile. If you find yourself lacking in your fat macros just add an avocado to your plate and you'll be good.
- Mushrooms – Depending on the type of mushrooms you are consuming you can get a healthy dose of vitamin C out of the deal. Sautee mushrooms with garlic and onion in grass-fed butter for a amazing keto-friendly snack. Watch the amount of garlic and onions you use as these veggies are higher in carbs.
- Eggs – As any fellow follower of keto knows, eggs are a staple low-carb food. The contain the perfect balance of protein and fat. You can eat eggs every day while on the keto diet. Feel free to be liberal in the amount you consume.
- Dark chocolate – Yes! You can have chocolate on the keto diet! You should stick to a 90 to 99% cocoa ratio. This form of chocolate is actually very good for you. Now, it is going to be quite bitter but you can consume chocolate that is sweetened by stevia and you'll feel as if you are eating a "regular" candy bar.
- Bone Broth – Bone broth is ultra-nourishing for the body. You can purchase it at the grocery store or easily make your own. When you start feeling symptoms of the keto flu,

warm yourself up a mug of bone broth and sip your symptoms away. Make sure to add pink Himalayan salt to the mix.

- Pork belly – Pork belly is fatty, delicious, and is what bacon is all about. Eat it with your eggs in the morning or make yourself a batch to snack on throughout the day. It is highly satiating.
- Berries – Although fruit is not ideal for a ketogenic diet, berries are. I don't want you to go overboard on them, but a handful of strawberries, blueberries, or blackberries here and there will do you no harm. They have a very low impact on the glycemic index. Plus, if you are feeling a craving for something sweet, berries can help satisfy the urge to reach for a donut.
- Grass-fed butter – You certainly may use corn-fed butter but grass-fed is the best. It tastes better and metabolizes differently within your body. Kerry Gold is an excellent brand to use. Yes, you can eat butter and lose weight. Imagine that!

When purchasing any foods, even the foods on the above list, it is very important to read labels. There are always going to be hidden carbs/sugars in certain foods that you never knew were there. For example, you purchase a bag of frozen strawberries and think you've got a glorious serving of nature's candy in your hand. You turn the bag over and see that the manufacturer added sugar to the berries to further sweeten them. Had you not checked you would have consumed added sugar and potentially kicked yourself out of ketosis.

Remember, you want to subtract the total carbs from the fiber content to know the net carbs that are in a food. Your goal is to keep it at 20 grams or less per day.

GETTING YOUR PANTRY PREPPED

You first need to determine whether you are a single or a family. This shouldn't be hard to determine, haha! If you are prepping for yourself, getting your pantry keto-ready is a bit simpler. However, if you are part of a family unit you need to either see if your family is able/wants to do keto with you or section off an area for your food.

When you have other people living with you and they aren't interested in keto you can't go tossing out all the carb-laden food. If you do that you're going to create a warzone within your home.

Prepping with a family will require more discipline on your part because you are going to have to live with non-keto foods in your home, however, I've done this myself and was successful. You can and will be successful, too!

So, as a family-prepper, if there are any carb-laden foods that are just yours, give them away. The same thing goes if you are single-prepper. If the food isn't half-eaten or spoiled, considering giving them to a family in need or donating to your local food pantry. There is no reason to throw away food that can help feed hungry bellies, no matter how carby it may be.

Once your pantry is cleared of non-keto foods, it is time to head to the grocery store. You can begin with the staple foods listed above or make your own low-carb list to work from. I like to sit down and look up keto recipes from some of my favorite keto websites. I'll then make a shopping list and meal plan for the week. Works like a charm! It always helps to have a list when going to the grocery store. You tell yourself that you are ONLY buying items from the list and you will not make any exceptions. This helps you to stay on task with keto-friendly foods. It also helps you stick to a budget.

TAKE A WALK AND GET A FEEL FOR WHICH RESTAURANT HAVE KETO OPTIONS

Or, you can drive, whichever tickles your fancy. I would opt for walking if possible because it is a way to get in some exercise.

Anyway...

You want to have a good idea of which eateries and cafes in your neighborhood are "safe zones" to eat at. Visit different establishments and ask them if you can have a menu. Scout the menu for keto-friendly options.

Honestly, I have found that every restaurant is going to have keto-options because you can MAKE them keto.

Let's say there is a small eatery that your family wants to go to and it sells primarily deep fried/battered food. Look for a chicken option. When you get your chicken you can simply peel away the breading and enjoy. Most places always have a side salad, too.

Did you know that fast food restaurants like McDonalds and Burger King allow you to order burgers without the bun? They'll typically warp your meat and toppings in a leaf of lettuce and give you a fork.

Now, don't get me wrong, you should not be eating like this all the time because these types of foods are not the healthiest but they will do when you're hungry and in a pinch.

4-WEEK BREAKDOWN OF BEGINNING YOUR KETO JOURNEY

WEEK 1

This is the starting point for your new keto journey. Congratulations! So, this week should feel pretty exciting for you. You'll undoubtedly be full of enthusiasm and drive. Perhaps, you may even experience a small twinge of fear because you've never done a low-carb diet before that requires you to eat lots of fat. That's okay and normal. I've experienced a bit of apprehension when I first started keto, myself.

As you begin to restrict carbohydrates you are most likely going to feel a lot of hunger pangs. In fact, you are going to crave carbs like crazy. This is normal. You see, most people are addicted to sugar. Yes, I said "addicted". So, like any addiction, there are going to be symptoms of withdrawal and cravings are one of them.

Tips to handle feelings of carb withdrawal and hunger:

- Add salt to your food as it replaces lost electrolytes and helps with dehydration. When you are thirsty you tend to have false food cravings. Make sure the salt is either sea or pink Himalayan. Mineral salt works well, too.
- Consume a tablespoon of coconut oil or MCT oil upon getting out of bed. This is pure, healthy fat that not only satiates your cravings but gives you an enormous burst of sustainable energy.
- Eat more butter! Butter is satiating and very nourishing for the body. Make sure you are consuming grass-fed if at all possible.
- Drink Bullet Proof Coffee (BPC) when hunger pangs strike. BPC is coffee made with MCT oil and butter. You place the hot coffee and oils in a blender and whip it into a frothy fat-filled drink that tastes absolutely lovely.
- When cravings strike, pop a few nuts in your mouth as they are known to help with hunger.
- Cheese is another great food to snack on when trying to beat the hunger beast.

Remember, keep cutting out the carbs and adding in good fats to your diet. Do not give in to your sugar cravings. All that will do is prolong your suffering and keep you stuck at square one.

WEEK 2

This is the week where you are going to probably see some results on the scale. Yay! Keep in mind that what you are seeing is not yet fat loss but water weight. When you restrict carbohydrates the stored glycogen in your fat cells is the first thing to leave your body. It comes out by way of water weight. You may even notice that you are urinating more during this week.

Now, if you aren't seeing any weight loss yet, that is also normal. Don't get upset or give up because your "whoosh" of water weight will surely come. Be patient and trust the process.

You may find yourself becoming familiar with the keto flu during week 2. Here are some tips to combating this pesky, but temporary, symptom:

- Make sure you are drinking an adequate amount of water and then drink some more.
- If you notice the keto flu is really being persistent, don't freak out. It just means your body is struggling to adapt to restricting carbs. This is normal, and many people experience a rough keto flu phase. It too shall pass.
- Make sure you are keeping your carbs at around 20 grams or less per day and following your fat macros. These things will help alleviate the keto flu.
- Make sure to follow all of your macros to avoid slipping into gluconeogenesis which will surely derail the fat burning train within your body.

Other physical symptoms that you may notice during week 2 are bad breath, cramps, fatigue, and waking up in the middle of the night to urinate. Here are some tips to help you deal with these symptoms:

- If you find that your breath isn't smelling all that fresh try chewing on mint leaves, taking a chlorophyll supplement, and regularly brushing your teeth and using a mouth rinse.
- Again, keep up with the salt intake so your electrolytes stay balanced. This will help with any cramps you are feeling. You may want to consider taking a magnesium/potassium supplement.
- If you are having trouble sleeping due to weird dreams, insomnia, and frequent urination, don't get upset. There are many people who deal with this when they start a low-carb diet. Sugar is seriously a beast to detox from and it does funny things to your body in the process. Try to not drink anything an hour before bed. Relax in a hot shower and turn off all screens and distraction before going to sleep for the night.
- Some folks complain of a "keto rash" especially in fat folds, groin area, and under the breasts. This is due to increased excretion of acetone and can be quite irritating. Use a powder or cornstarch on the areas until the rash clears up.

Remember, these symptoms are all temporary and will lessen and eventually disappear as you get deeper into your keto lifestyle.

WEEK 3

By now, you should be fairly acquainted with the daily needs of the keto diet. You'll find yourself having a good grasp on your macronutrient needs. In fact, you may feel as somewhat of a macro guru as you will begin to easily know the approximate amount of carbs, fats, and proteins in a meal. Look at you go!

Another great thing that comes with week 3 is your knowledge of knowing how to boost your fat intake whenever you feel that the day is passing and you are not getting your allotment. There is nothing wrong with adding a spoonful of butter or coconut oil to your food to increase your fat intake. At this point, you should have a "quick fat food" list in a handy place so you can easily utilize it.

WEEK 4

Hooray! You've soldiered on and reached week 4. Almost one month into your new keto WOE. That's awesome! At this point, for most people, the symptoms of the keto flu should be about gone. In fact, you are probably starting to feel pretty fine and dandy. I'm willing to bet the farm you are feeling more energized. Hiking up that steep hill has got nothing on you! Your focus is most likely better and you're reaping the benefits of mental clarity.

If you are not great around the kitchen, meaning, if you don't like to cook, your keto meals might be getting a bit repetitive at this point. Consider learning some new meals and being prepared with a stocked pantry of the items you need to make them. Weekly meal planning is quite helpful.

Lucky for you non-cook folks, this book is chock full of keto recipes and you are almost to that point. You'll find a meals for folks who are on-the-go and meals that take a more traditional cooking approach.

TROUBLESHOOTING COMMON ISSUES OF THE KETO DIET

So, you're not getting into ketosis. What are you doing wrong?

First of all, don't beat yourself up. You aren't "everyone". You are you. Some folks have a bit more of a struggle getting into ketosis than others and that's just life. However, there are a few questions to ask yourself:

"Am I watching my macros"?

"Am I watching for gluconeogenesis"?

"Am I watching for hidden carbs/sugars in my food?"

Please know that most people get into ketosis pretty quickly after 24 to 72 hours of carb restriction. You will most likely fall into this category.

What are net carbs and total carbs and which do you follow?

So, net carbs are carbs that are subtracted from the amount of natural fiber in a food. Many people use a net carb calculation because fiber is scientifically not a carbohydrate (25).

Total carbs is the number of carbs in a food that has not been subtracted by fiber or sugar alcohols. If you find yourself having trouble getting into ketosis, you can calculate your carb intake using the total number and then slowly switch back to the net carb method once you've been in ketosis for a while.

Is fat really good for you?

Yes. For years, we have been taught that fat makes you fat and saturated fat is basically the devil. This couldn't be further from the truth. Recent scientific studies have shown that fat is nourishing to the body and does not make you "fat". In fact, more research has shown that sugar makes you fat. When you combine fat and carbs together, this also makes you fat. Thus, that is why we've landed on the ketogenic diet.

If you are still concerned about saturated fats you can switch to eating only monounsaturated fats but let me warn you, this will significantly restrict the delicious foods you will be eating. Saturated fat is yummy and satiating.

Remember, keto is a high-fat diet and in order for it to work properly you need to consume your daily intake of fat.

Can you eat as much as you want?

Technically, yes. Keto is not a calorie counting type of diet. However, is also not a free-for-all, either. In the beginning, you may find yourself snacking on keto-approved foods all the time. This is normal. However, as you progress, you'll find you aren't as hungry as you were when eating a carb-heavy diet. In fact, most folks only eat 2 meals a day!

Try to stay within your macros and you'll be fine.

Why can't you eat 50 grams of carbs a day like Bob and still remain in ketosis?

Simply put, you aren't Bob. Everyone is different and has their own carb intake needs. You may only be able to tolerate 20 grams and Bob can tolerate 50 grams of carbs because of the state of metabolic damage that you are in.

There is a light at the end of the tunnel, though. The longer you remain in ketosis and eventually become fat adapted, you will be able to consume more carbs without being kicked out of ketosis.

Why haven't you lost weight yet?

If you haven't lost any weight, please don't stress about it. I'm willing to bet you have lost inches and your clothes fit better. Your body, at this point in time, may even be perfectly balanced and doesn't want to lose any weight.

Consider the health benefits you are seeing. Keto isn't all about weight loss, it's about getting your body out of a state of sugar addiction and becoming healthier over the long run.

Now, if it is obvious that you need to lose weight and you haven't done so yet, you may not fully be in ketosis, especially if your lack of weight loss is accompanied by constant keto flu symptoms.

Why is your cholesterol out of whack?

Many folks will see a significant increase in their cholesterol numbers when they first start keto. Both the HDL (good) and LDL (bad) tend to rise. I know this may worry you but it will even out and improve the longer you ar eon a ketogenic diet. When you see your cholesterol, especially the LDL, going up this signifies that your body is healing. Keep in mind that sugar is very inflammatory, and cholesterol is what tries to control the inflammation. Decreasing carbs is a shock to the system, initially, so the inflammation rises a bit. Depending on how bad your metabolic damage is, you may see a rise in cholesterol for a few months before it levels out.

YOU MADE IT! 1 MONTH IN TO KETO!

Congratulations! You have cleared your first month of keto. You craved carbs, combated the keto flu, and even saw weeks where the scale refused to move yet you kept ketoing on. Great for you!

You are now well prepped for the keto lifestyle and armed with a wealth of information.

This is the time where you need recipes to keep you going and not becoming bored with the basic keto foods you've been eating over the past 30 days. The recipes in the next chapter will help you to sustain your newfound ketogenic lifestyle.

Remember, if you have one of those days and eat a donut, dust yourself off, and realize it isn't the end of the world. You may fall out of ketosis for a short period of time but you can and will readapt quickly.

You've got this.

CHAPTER 4
All Planned Out And Ready!

<u>28 Day Meal Plan for Ketosis</u>

The ketogenic diet is an increasingly popular diet. So many people around the world have found success in weight loss through the keto lifestyle, and now you can too! The key to making this diet work is to monitor your macros carefully- the keto lifestyle consists of a diet that is high in fat, moderate in protein, and low in carbs. Because carbs are limited, it's also very important to keep your diet as nutritionally diverse as possible- this will ensure you're getting a balance of nutrients, in order to stay healthy and stick to this plan long term.

This meal plan will help you as you begin your journey into the keto lifestyle! For the next four weeks, you'll have your meals and snacks carefully planned out in order to provide you with a healthy, nutritionally diverse diet that adheres to the strict rules of the keto diet.

If you take a quick look at the meal plan, you'll see that every day includes three meals plus one snack, dessert, or drink to enjoy at your discretion. You'll also find that each recipe lists the calories and macros and that each day has a total. Remember, the meal plan is based on a daily intake of 1500 to 2,000 calories (give or take 100 calories) and an approximate macronutrient ratio of 70% to 80% fat, about 10% to 20% protein, and 5% to 10% carbohydrates.

In order to achieve ketosis, it's important to monitor carb intake carefully. Try to stay within 30 grams of net carbs a day (give or take a gram or two). Curious about the difference between gross carb count and net carb count? In order to easily calculate the net carbs in a recipe, subtract the insoluble fiber from the total carbohydrate and total fiber counts. Next, take a look at the sugar alcohol content- if the total count of sugar alcohols exceed 5 g, subtract half of that number from the total carb count to yield net carbs.

Protein intake is also quite important, and should be measured carefully. While some meal plans stress low protein intake, it's best to introduce yourself slowly to the keto lifestyle by keeping your protein in balance- you can still achieve ketosis with higher protein levels at first, and your body will naturally adjust to a point where it doesn't need or crave as much protein. You'll also find that your appetite will reduce the longer your body is in ketosis- this is a great sign! Listen to your body, and only eat as much as your body needs.

Intermittent fasting is a great way to jolt your body into ketosis, and one of the cornerstones of the keto lifestyle. While this meal plan provides you with food options daily, feel free to fast one day a week if you're able to, or skip a meal here and there in order to introduce yourself to the concept. While fasting, remember to consume plenty of water, and help yourself to a cup of bone broth if you're feeling hungry.

Pay close attention to the shopping list- as you may have noticed, we've given you a few substitution options. While the majority of these items can all be found in grocery and health food stores, we wanted to ensure that you had viable alternative options in the event you can't find something. Each of the substitution options listed can be used in the exact same quantity and application as the original ingredient item.

To save you time and money, some of the protein and produce items are can also be carried over into the following week- for example, if you only need 4 oz of chicken in one week, but 8 oz the week after, it makes sense to purchase it all in one shot. Remember with meat especially, it's usually less expensive to purchase in bulk and portion and freeze it to be used over a longer period of time.

Without further ado, here are EIGHT 7-day meal plans to get you started!

TRADITIONAL MEAL PLAN

This meal plan is for folks who have time to cook and like to be in the kitchen. Of course, it is for everyone else, too. You'll find the recipes to be concise and easy to make. Plus, these meals are totally delicious if I do say so myself!

Save time and money on your keto diet by doing the following:

- Intermittent fasting- If you're not hungry, don't eat! While this may seem like a simple enough premise, it is something to keep in mind as intermittent fasting aids in raising your ketone levels. The recipes and meal recommendations in this guide are here to give you options as you begin your keto journey, but don't feel obligated to eat just because the plan is telling you to do so (LISTEN to your body!)

- Meal prep- Look over your meal plan every week, as well as your shopping list, and figure out what you can prep ahead of time to save yourself time during the week. Many of these recipes can be prepped ahead of time and kept on hand to enjoy at your convenience. Dinner leftovers make fast, easy lunches, and breakfast can be a repeat of your favourite recipe (if you love keto lattes in the morning, stick with that!)

- The recipes in this plan are made to empower you to make your own food choices! Particularly in the dinner section (because, let's face it- dinner is usually the one meal we all struggle with!), you will find an assortment of side dish recipes that are meant to be eaten in conjunction with a protein, and usually one or two other sides as well. The meal plan is a guideline, but as you become more comfortable with it, feel free to make small swaps here and there as you see fit (just make sure to track the macros!)

- Many of these recipes come with add-on options (such as added sour cream in the quesadillas recipe), with individual macros listed below the overall nutritional info. If you choose to use the add-on items, make sure to adjust the macros as needed.

Week 1 Traditonal Meal Plan					
Day	**Breakfast**	**Lunch**	**Dinner**	**Snack/Dessert**	**Calories/Macros**
1	Cheesy Scrambled Eggs 424 cal 39.8 fat 15.3 protein 1.9 carbs	Salmon, spinach and goat cheese Salad 311 cal 17.5 g fat 24 g protein 11 g carbs	4 oz Baked Salmon with warm mushrooms and brown butter 650 cal 54 g fat 40 g protein 6 g carbs	2 oz macadamia nuts 241 cal 25,4 g fat 2.7 g protein 1 g carbs	Calories: 1626 Fat: 136.7 g Protein: 82 g Net Carbs: 19.9 g
2	Dairy Free Keto Pumpkin Spice Latte 190 cal 18 g fat 6 g protein 0.9 g carbs	Green Goddess Avo Salad 905 cal 75.5 g fat 32 g protein 10 g carbs	Eggplant Parmesan 385 cal 28.1 g fat 22.5 g protein 12.3 g carbs	FASTING PERIOD Intermittent fasting is a cornerstone of the keto diet, and helps your body achieve ketosis (water allowed)	Calories: 1480 Fat: 121.6 g Protein: 60.5 g Net Carbs: 23.2 g

3	Greek Style Scrambled Eggs 404 cal 37.8 g fat 15.3 g protein 1.9 g carbs	Eggplant Parmesan (leftover) 385 cal 28.1 g fat 22.5 g protein 12.3 g carbs	4 oz Steak (cooked to your liking) with Cauliflower Goat Cheese Mash 785 cal 60.1 g fat 56 g protein 4.6 g carbs	FASTING PERIOD Intermittent fasting is a cornerstone of the keto diet, and helps your body achieve ketosis (water allowed)	Calories: 1574 Fat:126 g Protein: 93.8 g Net Carbs: 18.8 g
4	Western Scrambled Eggs 498 cal 43.8g fat 23.4g protein 2,9 g carbs	Beef and Avocado Lettuce Wraps 454 cal 37 fat 21 protein 6 carbs	1 serving lemon and thyme chicken legs with 1 serving Bacon Parmesan Asparagus 639 cal 61.8 g fat 65.6 protein 6.6 g carbs	4 stalks celery, ¼ bell pepper and 1 serving Tahini 89 cal 8 g fat 2.6 g protein 1 g carb	Calories: 1680 Fat: 150.6 g Protein: 112.6 g Net Carbs: 16.5 g
5	Bacon Egg and Avo Sandwich 899 cal 83.9 g fat 24.2 g protein 4.1 g carbs	1 serving lemon and thyme chicken legs with 1 cup greens, ½ oz pecans, and 1 serving Strawberry Balsamic Dressing 599 cal 53 g fat 30,5 g protein 0.9 g carbs	Bacon Wrapped Cod 323 cal 27.6 fat 17.5 protein 0.7 carbs	FASTING PERIOD Intermittent fasting is a cornerstone of the keto diet, and helps your body achieve ketosis (water allowed)	Calories: 1821 Fat: 164.5 g Protein: 72.2 g Net Carbs: 18.8 g

6	Coconut Chia Pudding 451 cal 42 g fat 6.6 g protein 8 g carbs	Leftover Bacon Wrapped Cod with 1 serving Bacon Parmesan Asparagus 583 cal 54.4 fat 52.6 protein 6.7 carbs	Pesto Chicken Casserole 501 cal 37.6 g fat 38 g protein 4.6 g carbs	1 oz pecans 197 cal 23.3 g fat 3 g protein 1.1 g carbs	Calories: 1732 Fat 157.3 g Protein: 100.2 g Net Carbs: 20.4 g
7	Dairy Free Mocha Latte 190 cal 18 g fat 6 g protein 0.9 g carbs	Eggplant Parmesan (leftover) 385 cal 28.1 g fat 22.5 g protein 12.3 g carbs	4 oz Steak (cooked to your liking) with Cauliflower Goat Cheese Mash and Bacon Parmesan Asparagus 1045 cal 86.9 g fat 91.1 g protein 10.6 g carbs	FASTING PERIOD Intermittent fasting is a cornerstone of the keto diet, and helps your body achieve ketosis (water allowed)	Calories: 1620 Fat 133 g Protein:119.6 g Net Carbs: 23.8 g

Week 2 Traditional Meal Plan

Day	Breakfast	Lunch	Dinner	Snack/Dessert	Calories/Macros
8	Double Egg Breakfast Sandwich 607 cal 53 fat 30,2 protein 2.4 carbs	Keto Quesadillas 330 cal 21.5 fat 29.7 protein 4.1 carbs	Southwest Chicken Chili 410 cal 23.1 fat 28.9 protein 7 carbs	Coconut Chia Pudding 451 cal 42 g fat 6.6 g protein 8 g carbs	Calories: 1798 Fat: 139.6 g Protein: 95.4 g Net Carbs: 22.5 g
9	Strawberry Smoothie with 1 Breakfast Roll and 1 tbsp almond butter 737 cal 53 fat 33.5 g protein 8.3 g net carbs	Southwest Chicken Chili (leftover) 410 cal 23.1 fat 28.9 protein 7 carbs	Asian Style Beef Salad 603 cal 22 g fat 85.2 g protein 5 g carbs	FASTING PERIOD Intermittent fasting is a cornerstone of the keto diet, and helps your body achieve ketosis (water allowed)	Calories: 1750 Fat: 98.1 g Protein: 147.6 g Net Carbs: 20.3 g
10	1 serving Cinnamon Roll Donuts 160 cal 11.8 g fat 3.2 g protein 1.2 g carbs	Asian Style Beef Salad (leftover) 603 cal 22 g fat 85.2 g protein 5 g carbs	Middle Eastern Halloumi 700 cal 53.2 g fat 33.7 g protein 15 g carbs	Coconut Matcha Latte 255 cal 28.8 g fat 3.4 g protein 3 g carbs	Calories: 1718 Fat: 115.8 g Protein: 125.3 g Net Carbs: 24.2 g

11	Dairy Free Keto Latte 190 cal 18 fat 6 g protein 0.9 g carbs	Italian Chopped Salad 790 cal 66 g fat 47 protein 5.9 carbs	Coconut Curry Shiratake Noodles 557 cal 41.7 g fat 33.7 g protein 13 g carbs	1 serving Cinnamon Roll Donuts 160 cal 11.8 g fat 3.2 g protein 1.2 g carbs	Calories: 1697 Fat: 137.5 g Protein: 89.9 g Net Carbs: 21 g
12	Goat Cheese Pancakes 425 cal 39 fat 14 protein 5 carbs	Coconut Curry Shiratake Noodles (leftover) 557 cal 41.7 g fat 33.7 g protein 13 g carbs	Lemon and Thyme Chicken Leg with Mushrooms and Brown Butter (plus optional side of greens) 879 cal 74.8 g fat 48.5 g protein 6 g carbs	FASTING PERIOD Intermittent fasting is a cornerstone of the keto diet, and helps your body achieve ketosis (water allowed)	Calories: 1861 Fat: 155.5 g Protein: 96.2 g Net Carbs: 24 g
13	Keto Dairy Free Vanilla Latte 190 cal 18 g fat 6 g protein 0.9 g carbs	Lemon and Thyme Chicken Leg with Mushrooms and Brown Butter (Left over) With ½ cup greens 879 cal 74.8 g fat 48.5 g protein 6 g carbs	Creamy Bacon and Spinach Zucchini Noodles 770 cal 65 fat 37.6 protein 12 g carbs	FASTING PERIOD Intermittent fasting is a cornerstone of the keto diet, and helps your body achieve ketosis (water allowed)	Calories: 1839 Fat: 157.8 g Protein: 92.1 g Net Carbs:18.9 g

| 14 | Keto Dairy Free Pumpkin Spice Latte plus 1 egg cooked to your liking 235 cal 23 g fat 11.5 g protein 0.9 g carbs | Creamy Bacon and Spinach Zucchini Noodles 770 cal 65 fat 37.6 protein 12 g carbs | Taco Night 860 cal 77.6 fat 54.5 protein 3.9 carbs | FASTING PERIOD Intermittent fasting is a cornerstone of the keto diet, and helps your body achieve ketosis (water allowed) | Calories: 1865 Fat: 165.6 g Protein: 103.6 g Net Carbs: 16.8 g |

Week 3 Traditional Meal Plan

Day	Breakfast	Lunch	Dinner	Snack/Dessert	Calories/Macros
15	Western Scrambled Eggs 498 cal 43.8 g fat 23.4 g protein 2.9 g carbs	Burrito Bowl (using leftover taco meat) 545 calories 32 g fat 48.6 g protein 11 g carbs	Keto Cabbage Rolls 405 cal 16.4 g fat 53.6 g protein 7 g carbs	2 oz Almonds 328 cal 28.4 g fat 12 g protein 4 g carb	Calories: 1776 Fat:120.6 g Protein:137.6 g Net Carbs: 24.9 g
16	Halloumi Shakshouka with Keto Dairy Free Vanilla Latte 350 cal 29.8 g fat 9.2 g protein 2.1 g carbs	Keto Cabbage Rolls (left over) 405 cal 16.4 g fat 53.6 g protein 7 g carbs	Asian Style Beef Salad 603 cal 22 g fat 85.2 g protein 5 g carbs	3 oz prosciutto with 2 oz mozzarella 283 cal 14.8 g fat 33.6 g protein 3 g carb	Calories: 1641 Fat: 83 g Protein: 181.6 g Net Carbs: 18.1 g

17	Dairy Free Mocha Latte 190 cal 18 g fat 6 g protein 0.9 g carbs	Asian Style Beef Salad (leftover) 603 cal 22 g fat 85.2 g protein 5 g carbs	Bacon Wrapped Cod with Mushrooms and Brown Butter, and Bacon Parmesan Asparagus 1083 cal 101.4 g fat 70.6 g protein 12.7 carbs	FASTING PERIOD Intermittent fasting is a cornerstone of the keto diet, and helps your body achieve ketosis (water allowed)	Calories: 1876 Fat: 141.4 g Protein: 161.8 g Net Carbs: 18.5 g
18	Strawberry Smoothie 150 cal 14 fat 0.1 g protein 1.4 g net carbs	Bacon wrapped cod with ½ cup greens and bacon parmesan asparagus 626 cal 54.4 g fat 52.6 g protein 6.7 g carbs	Shiratake Carbonara 720 cal 67 g fat 33.9 g protein 4.7 g carb	Coconut Matcha Latte 255 cal 28.8 g fat 3.4 g protein 3 g carbs	Calories: 1751 Fat:164.2 g Protein: 89.1 g Net Carbs: 15.8 g
19	Greek Style Scrambled Eggs 404 cal 37.8 fat 15.3 protein 1.9 carbs	Keto Cabbage Rolls (leftover) 405 cal 16.4 g fat 53.6 g protein 7 g carbs	Roulade of Chicken 700 cal 63.8 g fat 72.9 g protein 3.6 g carbs	FASTING PERIOD Intermittent fasting is a cornerstone of the keto diet, and helps your body achieve ketosis (water allowed)	Calories: 1509 Fat: 112.8 g Protein: 90.5 g Net Carbs: 21.3 g
20	Dairy Free Keto Pumpkin Spice Latte 190 cal 18 g fat 6 g protein 0.9 g carbs	1 serving Chicken Roulade (leftovers) with ½ cup spinach and 1 serving Creamy Poppy seed dressing 937 cal 90.6 fat 73.9 protein 4.6 g carbs	Keto Pizza 761 cal 52 g fat 70 g protein 7 carbs	FASTING PERIOD Intermittent fasting is a cornerstone of the keto diet, and helps your body achieve ketosis (water allowed)	Calories: 1888 Fat: 160.6 g Protein: 149.9 g Net Carbs: 12.5 g

Day					
21	Smoked salmon, cream cheese and greens breakfast sandwich 539 cal 53 g fat 35.6 g protein 5.7 g carbs	Keto Cabbage Rolls (leftover) 405 cal 16.4 g fat 53.6 g protein 7 g carbs	4 oz steak with Cauliflower Goat Cheese Mash 785 cal 59.8 g fat 56 g protein 4.6 g net carb	FASTING PERIOD Intermittent fasting is a cornerstone of the keto diet, and helps your body achieve ketosis (water allowed)	Calories: 1729 Fat: 129.2 g Protein:145.2 g Net Carbs: 17.3 g

Week 4 Traditional Meal Plan

Day	Breakfast	Lunch	Dinner	Snack/Dessert	Calories/Macros
22	Double Egg Sandwich 607 cal 53 g fat 30.2 g protein 2.4 g carbs	Keto Quesadillas with 3 tbsp sour cream 407 cal 29.1 g fat 30.8 g protein 5.6 g carbs	Shiratake Carbonara (leftover) 720 cal 67 g fat 33.9 g protein 4.7 g carb	4 stalks celery, ¼ bell pepper and 1 serving Tahini 89 cal 8 g fat 2.6 g protein 1 g carb	Calories: 1823 Fat: 157.1 g Protein: 97.5 g Net Carbs:13.7 g
23	Swiss Omelette 425 cal 39 g fat 14 g protein 5 g carbs	Keto Pizza (leftover) 761 cal 52 g fat 70 g protein 7 carbs	1 serving lemon and thyme chicken legs with 1 serving Bacon Parmesan Asparagus 639 cal 61.8 g fat 65.6 protein 6.6 g carbs	FASTING PERIOD Intermittent fasting is a cornerstone of the keto diet, and helps your body achieve ketosis (water allowed)	Calories: 1825 Fat: 152.8 g Protein: 149.6 g Net Carbs: 18.6 g

24	Cheesy Chicken Breakfast Burrito 830 cal 75.2 g fat 50.3 g protein 3.5 g carbs	½ cup greens with 2 strips bacon and 1 serving Creamy Onion Poppyseed dressing 446 cal 42.7 g fat 15.5 g protein 1.7 g carbs	Pesto Chicken Casserole 501 cal 37.6 g fat 38 g protein 4.6 g carbs	FASTING PERIOD Intermittent fasting is a cornerstone of the keto diet, and helps your body achieve ketosis (water allowed)	Calories: 1777 Fat: 155.5 g Protein: 103.8 g Net Carbs: 9.8 g
25	Mushroom, Spinach and Goat Cheese Frittata 316 cal 27 fat 16.4 protein 2.4 carbs	Italian Chopped Salad 790 cal 66 g fat 47 g protein 5.9 g carbs	Oysters Rockefeller with optional side of greens 700 cal 55.6g fat 60.9 g protein 13 g carbs	FASTING PERIOD Intermittent fasting is a cornerstone of the keto diet, and helps your body achieve ketosis (water allowed)	Calories: 1806 Fat: 148.6 g Protein: 119 g Net Carbs: 21.3 g
26	Dairy Free Keto Mocha Latte 190 calories 18 g fat 6g protein 0.9 g carbs	Leftover Mushroom, Spinach and Goat Cheese Frittata with ½ cup greens and 1 serving Strawberry Balsamic Dressing 536 cal 52 fat 16.4 protein 2.7 carbs	Coconut Curry Shirataki noodles with 1 serving Lemon and Thyme Chicken (leftover) 936 cal 69.5 g fat 64.2 g protein 13 g carbs	FASTING PERIOD Intermittent fasting is a cornerstone of the keto diet, and helps your body achieve ketosis (water allowed)	Calories: 1662 Fat: 139.5 g Protein: 86.6 g Net Carbs: 16.6 g

27	Cheesy Scrambled Eggs 424 cal 39.8g fat 15.3 g protein 1.9 g carbs	Pesto Chicken Casserole (leftover) 501 cal 37.6 g fat 38 g protein 4.6 g carbs	Pork Chops with Mushrooms 805 cal 73.4g fat 45.6 g protein 3.4 g carb	FASTING PERIOD Intermittent fasting is a cornerstone of the keto diet, and helps your body achieve ketosis (water allowed)	Calories: 1730 Fat: 150.8 g Protein: 98.9 g Net Carbs: 10.9 g
28	Double Egg Breakfast Sandwich 607 cal 53g fat 30.2 g protein 2.4 g carbs	Pork Chops with Mushrooms (leftover) 805 cal 73.4g fat 45.6 g protein 3.4 g carb	Eggplant Parmesan 385 cal 28.1 g fat 22.5 g protein 12.3 g carbs	FASTING PERIOD Intermittent fasting is a cornerstone of the keto diet, and helps your body achieve ketosis (water allowed)	Calories: 1797 Fat: 154.5 g Protein: 98.3g Net Carbs: 18.1 g

QUICK KETO MEAL PLAN

If you're a busy bee and don't have a lot of time to spend in the kitchen or on prep work, this quick keto meal plan will work wonders for you and your schedule. Get ready to be wowed with food, my friend.

Week 1 Quick Meal Plan					
Day	Breakfast	Lunch	Dinner	Snack/Dessert	Calories/Macros
1	Blue Smoothie 189 cal 16.6 fat 3.1 protein 1 carbs	Loaded Avocado Salad 430 cal 35.5 g fat 13.2 g protein 8 g carbs	3 oz Baked Salmon with leftover Loaded Avocado Salad 540 cal 41 g fat 29.7 g protein 8 g carbs	Caprese Rolls with Prosciutto 95 cal 4 g fat 12.5 g protein 1 g carbs	Calories: 1254 Fat: 149.9 g Protein: 58.5 g Net Carbs: 18 g

2	Coconut smoothie bowl 726 cal 69.4 g fat 11.4 g protein 6 g carbs	Keto Lunchables 590 cal 37.6 g fat 28.6 g protein 6 g carbs.	Lettuce Wrapped Chicken Fajitas 320 cal 20 g fat 26.2 g protein 4 g carbs	FASTING PERIOD Intermittent fasting is a cornerstone of the keto diet, and helps your body achieve ketosis (water allowed)	Calories: 1636 Fat: 127 g Protein: 66.2 g Net Carbs: 16 g
3	Microwave Scrambled Eggs 394 cal 35.7 g fat 17.4 g protein 0.1 g carbs	Salmon and Avocado Nori Rolls 380 cal 29.6 g fat 20.6 g protein 3.5 g carbs	Coconut Lime Noodles and Tofu 303 cal 14.2 g fat 28.9 g protein 9.1 g carbs	2 oz pecans 390 calories 40 g fat 6 g protein 2 g carbs	Calories: 1467 Fat: 119.5 g Protein: 72.9 g Net Carbs: 14.7 g
4	Green Smoothie 350 cal 34g fat 4.1 g protein 1.5 g carbs	1 serving Cream of Broccoli Soup with easy green salad 478 cal 47 fat 3.3 protein 3.1 carbs	Cheesy Chicken Bake 488 cal 22.3 g fat 34 protein 9.3 g carbs	Beef Broth 273cal 28.6 g fat 4.9 g protein 0.9 g carbs	Calories: 1589 Fat: 131.9 g Protein: 46.3 g Net Carbs: 14.8 g

5	Microwave Scrambled Eggs with your choice of inclusions* 394 cal 35.7 g fat 17.4 g protein 0.1 g carbs *Macros will vary slightly dependent upon inclusions	Leftover Coconut Lime Noodles 303 cal 14.2 g fat 28.9 g protein 9.1 g carbs	1 serving Cream of Broccoli Soup With Easy Green Salad 478 cal 51.1 fat 3.3 protein 3.1 carbs	2 Servings Almond Coconut Fat Bomb 400 cal 40 g fat 6 g protein 4 g carbs	Calories: 1575 Fat: 141 g Protein: 55.6 g Net Carbs: 16.3 g
6	Nut Butter Smoothie Bowl 183 cal 13.3 fat 8.6 protein 0.1 carbs	Thai Chicken Salad 303 cal 14.2 fat 28.3 protein 9.1 carbs	Avocado BLT 540 cal 46.1 g fat 18.3 g protein 5.6 g carbs	Veggie Sticks and Tahini 89 cal 8 g fat 2.6 g protein 1 g carb	Calories: 1591 Fat 146.4 g Protein: 36.2 g Net Carbs: 10.8 g
7	Chicken Parm Fritatta 600 cal 31 g fat 45 g protein 9.3 g carbs	FASTING PERIOD Intermittent fasting (water allowed) *Note- if you don't think you can make it through the day without lunch, have your snack here and fast later	Salmon Putanesca 600 cal 30.3 g fat 72.4 g protein 8 g net carbs	2 servings Guacamole Deviled Eggs 390 cal 34 g fat 14 g protein 6 g carbs	Calories: 1590 Fat 95.3 g Protein:131.4 g Net Carbs: 23.3 g

Week 2 Quick Meal Plan

Day	Breakfast	Lunch	Dinner	Snack/Dessert	Calories/Macros
8	Blue Smoothie 189 cal 16.6 fat 3.1 protein 1 carbs	Salmon Putanesca with Easy Green Salad 846 cal 50.6 fat 72.8 protein 8.1 carbs	Ham and Swiss Cheese Crustless Quiche 566 cal 43.2 fat 36.3 protein 5.6 carbs	Coconut Matcha Fat Bomb 100 cal 11.5 g fat 0.2 g protein 2 g carbs	Calories: 1701 Fat: 121.9 g Protein: 112.4 g Net Carbs: 16.7 g
9	Leftover Ham and Swiss Crustless Quiche 566 cal 43.2 fat 36.3 protein 5.6 carbs	Tuna Salad Lettuce Wraps 466 cal 24.2 g fat 48.1 g protein 7.1 g net carbs	Chicken a la king 494 cal 36.9 g fat 29.1 g protein 4.3 g carbs	Beef Broth 273cal 28.6 g fat 4.9 g protein 0.9 g carbs	Calories: 1799 Fat:132.9 g Protein: 118.4 g Net Carbs: 17.9 g
10	Matcha Smoothie Bowl 691 cal 67.9 g fat 12.9 g protein 8 g carbs	Cream of Broccoli Soup 232 cal 22.8 fat 2.9 protein 3 carbs	Portobello Burger 485 cal 30 fat 48.6 protein 2 carbs	Caprese Rolls with Prosciutto 95 cal 4 g fat 12.5 g protein 1 g carbs	Calories: 1503 Fat: 124.7 g Protein: 76.9 g Net Carbs: 14 g
11	Green Smoothie 350 cal 34 fat 4.1 g protein 1.5 g carbs	Caprese Salad 534 cal 52.2fat 16.6 protein 3 carbs	Thai Chicken Salad 303 cal 14.2 g fat 28.9 g protein 9.1 g carbs	2 Servings Almond Coconut Fat Bomb 400 cal 40 g fat 6 g protein 4 g carbs	Calories: 1587 Fat: 140.4 g Protein: 55.6 g Net Carbs: 17.6 g

12	Easy Eggs Benedict 366 cal 32.8 fat 11.5 protein 5 carbs	Keto Lunchables with your choice of inclusions 590 cal 37.6 g fat 28.6 g protein 6 g carbs	Shrimp Stir Fry 600 cal 56g fat 30.6 g protein 7 g carbs	FASTING PERIOD Intermittent fasting is a cornerstone of the keto diet, and helps your body achieve ketosis (water allowed)	Calories: 1556 Fat: 126.4 g Protein: 70.7 g Net Carbs:18 g
13	Microwave Scrambled Eggs with your choice of inclusions 394 cal 35.7 g fat 17.4 g protein 0.1 g carbs	Leftover Shrimp Stir Fry 600 cal 56g fat 30.6 g protein 7 g carbs	Middle Eastern Style Stuffed Tomatoes 400 cal 33 fat 22.9 protein 5 g carbs	2 servings Coconut Matcha Fat Bombs 200 cal 23 g fat 0.4 g protein 4 g carbs	Calories: 1594 Fat: 147.7 g Protein: 71.3 g Net Carbs: 16.1 g
14	Nutty Coffee Plus 3 Pieces Bacon 476 calories 39.6 g fat 26.6 g protein 2.1 carbs	Leftover Middle Eastern Stuffed Tomatoes 400 cal 33 fat 22.9 protein 5 g carbs	Ma Po Tofu 449 cal 30.1 fat 35.1 protein 6 carbs	Caprese Rolls with Prosciutto 95 cal 4 g fat 12.5 g protein 1 g carbs	Calories: 1420 Fat: 106.7 g Protein: 97.1 g Net Carbs: 14.1 g

Week 3 Quick Meal Plan

Day	Breakfast	Lunch	Dinner	Snack/Dessert	Calories/Macros
15	Scotch Eggs 442 cal 46 g fat 25 g protein 0 g carbs	Easy green salad with 4 oz baked salmon 396 calories 35.3 g fat 22.4 g protein 0.1 g carbs	Bacon-butter cod with parmesan crusted cauliflower 273 cal 20 g fat 23 g protein 2 g carbs	2 oz Almonds 328 cal 28.4 g fat 12 g protein 4 g carb	Calories: 1439 Fat:129.7 g Protein: 82.4 g Net Carbs: 6.1 g
16	Keto Lemon Tea Plus 1 egg any way and 3 pieces bacon 622 cal 55.6 g fat 27.3 g protein 4.2 g carbs	Leftover Butter-Bacon Cod with parmesan crusted cauliflower 273 cal 20 g fat 23 g protein 2 g carbs	Cheesy Mushrooms with easy green salad 370 cal 43.8 g fat 1.9 g protein 0.3 g carbs	Beef Broth 273cal 28.6 g fat 4.9 g protein 0.9 g carbs	Calories: 1538 Fat: 141 g Protein: 57.1 g Net Carbs: 7.4 g
17	Coconut Smoothie 638 cal 57.4 g fat 7.2 g protein 9 g carbs	Leftover Cheesy Mushroom with Easy green salad 370 cal 43.8 fat 1.9 g protein 0.3 carbs	Cream of Broccoli Soup 232 cal 22.8 fat 2.9 protein 3 carbs	Veggie Sticks and Guacamole 294 cal 30 g fat 12 g protein 4.2 g carbs	Calories: 1534 Fat: 154 g Protein: 24 g Net Carbs: 26.4 g

18	Easy Eggs Benedict 366 cal 32.8 fat 11.5 protein 5 carbs	Chicken BLT Salad 734 cal 52.5 g fat 45.1 g protein 9 g carbs	Bacon-Tomato-Cheddar Soup 270 cal 21.9 g fat 12.2 g protein 1 g carb	2 servings Prosciutto Mozzarella and Basil rolls 190 calories 8 g fat 25 g protein 2 g carbs	Calories: 1560 Fat: 115.2 g Protein: 93.8 g Net Carbs: 17 g
19	Blue Smoothie plus 1 egg and 3 slices bacon 560 cal 44.8 fat 29.8 protein 2.2 carbs	Thai Chicken Salad 303 cal 14.2 fat 28.3 protein 9.1 carbs	Pesto Pasta 646 cal 53.8 g fat 32.4 g protein 10 g carbs	FASTING PERIOD Intermittent fasting is a cornerstone of the keto diet, and helps your body achieve ketosis (water allowed)	Calories: 1509 Fat: 112.8 g Protein: 90.5 g Net Carbs: 21.3 g
20	Keto Lemon Tea 251 cal 27.4 g fat 0.6 g protein 3 g carbs	Leftover pesto pasta 646 cal 53.8 g fat 32.4 g protein 10 g carbs	Cheesy Meatballs 331 cal 20.6 g fat 40.1 g protein 10 carbs	2 oz pecans 390 calories 40 g fat 6 g protein 2 g carbs	Calories: 1618 Fat: 141.8 g Protein: 79.4 g Net Carbs: 25 g
21	Microwave Scrambled Eggs with choice of inclusions 394 cal 35.7 g fat 17.4 g protein 0.1 g carbs	Leftover Cheesy Meatballs 331 cal 20.6 g fat 40.1 g protein 10 carbs	Chicken, spinach and goat cheese salad 700 cal 51.8 g fat 45.3 g protein 3 g net carb	Beef Broth 273cal 28.6 g fat 4.9 g protein 0.9 g carbs	Calories: 1698 Fat: 136.7 g Protein: 107.7 g Net Carbs: 14 g

Week 4 Quick Meal Plan

Day	Breakfast	Lunch	Dinner	Snack/Dessert	Calories/Macros
22	Green Smoothie 350 cal 34g fat 4.1 g protein 1.5 g carbs	Southwest Chicken Avocado Salad 800 cal 53.1 g fat 41.9 g protein 5 g carbs	Bacon-Tomato-Cheddar Soup 270 cal 21.9 g fat 12.2 g protein 1 g carb	Caprese Rolls with Prosciutto 95 cal 4 g fat 12.5 g protein 1 g carbs	Calories: 1515 Fat: 113 g Protein: 70.7 g Net Carbs: 8.5 g
23	Keto Lemon Tea 251 cal 27.4 g fat 0.6 g protein 3 g carbs	Easy green salad with 4 oz baked salmon 396 calories 35.3 g fat 22.4 g protein 0.1 g carbs	Baked Cod with lemony asparagus 554 cal 26 g fat 81 g protein 1.3 g carbs	2 servings Coconut Matcha Fat Bombs 200 cal 23 g fat 0.4 g protein 4 g carbs	Calories: 1401 Fat: 111.7 g Protein: 111.4 g Net Carbs: 8.4 g
24	Asparagus and Goat Cheese Omelette 694 cal 59.7 g fat 35 g protein 4.5 g carbs	Leftover Baked Cod with lemony asparagus 554 cal 26 g fat 81 g protein 1.3 g carbs	Bacon-Tomato-Cheddar Soup 270 cal 21.9 g fat 12.2 g protein 1 g carb	Veggie Sticks and Tahini 89 cal 8 g fat 2.6 g protein 1 g carb	Calories: 1607 Fat: 115.6 g Protein: 130.8 g Net Carbs: 7.8 g

25	Easy Eggs Benedict 366 cal 32.8 fat 11.5 protein 5 carbs	Keto Lunchables with your choice of inclusions 590 cal 37.6 g fat 28.6 g protein 6 g carbs	Shrimp Stir Fry 600 cal 56g fat 30.6 g protein 7 g carbs	FASTING PERIOD Intermittent fasting is a cornerstone of the keto diet, and helps your body achieve ketosis (water allowed)	Calories: 1556 Fat:76.4 g Protein: 70.7 g Net Carbs: 18 g
26	Nutty Coffee 168 calories 15.8 g fat 5.5g protein 2.1 carbs	Leftover Shrimp Stir Fry 600 cal 56g fat 30.6 g protein 7 g carbs	Asparagus, goat cheese and smoked salmon salad 466 cal 31.6 g fat 41.9 g protein 2.3 g carbs	2 servings Guacamole Deviled Eggs 390 cal 34 g fat 14 g protein 6 g carbs	Calories: 1624 Fat: 117.4 g Protein: 92 g Net Carbs: 17.4 g
27	Matcha Smoothie Bowl 691 cal 67.9 g fat 12.9 g protein 8 g carbs	Easy green salad with 4 oz baked salmon 396 calories 35.3 g fat 22.4 g protein 0.1 g carbs	Bacon-Tomato-Cheddar Soup 270 cal 21.9 g fat 12.2 g protein 1 g carb	1 serving coconut matcha fat bombs 100 cal 10.3 g fat 0.2 g protein 2 g net carbs	Calories: 1457 Fat: 135.4 g Protein: 47.7 g Net Carbs: 11.1 g
28	Southwest style eggs 546 cal 35 g fat 26 g protein 12 g carbs	Chicken and Avocado Nori Wraps 657 cal 50.5 g fat 33 g protein 9 g carbs	Baked Cod with lemony asparagus 554 cal 26 g fat 81 g protein 1.3 g carbs	Veggie Sticks and Tahini 89 cal 8 g fat 2.6 g protein 1 g carb	Calories: 1846 Fat: 119.5 g Protein: 142.6 g Net Carbs: 23.3 g

CHAPTER 5
Oh Something's Cookin

Breakfast

Cheesy Scrambled Eggs ✓

Scrambled eggs and cheese are the ultimate comfort food.

Serving: 1

Serving Size: whole recipe

Prep Time: 5 minutes

Cook Time: >5 minutes

Ingredients

2 eggs, beaten

1 oz butter

1 oz shredded cheddar cheese

Instructions

Beat the eggs with a pinch of salt and pepper.

Preheat a small pan over medium heat, and melt in the butter

Pour in the eggs, and stir constantly for 3 minutes, until cooked through

Add in the cheese, and stir for another minute.

Nutrition: 424 calories, 39.8 g fat, 15.3 g protein, 1.9 g net carbs

Strawberry Smoothie

This smoothie is so easy to make, and a low calorie way to start your morning. Enjoy on its own, or as a beverage with your favourite breakfast food. It also makes a great snack any time of the day!

Serving: 1

Serving Size: whole recipe

Prep Time: 5 minutes

Cook Time: 0 minutes

Ingredients

2 frozen strawberries, thawed slightly

¾ almond milk

¼ tsp erythritol (optional)

1 tbsp coconut oil

Instructions

Blend together all ingredients until smooth. Serve immediately.

Nutrition: 150 calories, 14 g fat, 0.1 g protein, 1.4 g net carbs

Greek Style Scrambled Eggs

These eggs are creamy, delicious, and have a yummy mediterranean twist!

Serving: 1

Serving Size: whole recipe

Prep Time: 5 minutes

Cook Time: >5 minutes

Ingredients

2 eggs, beaten

1 tsp dried oregano

1 oz butter

1 oz feta

Instructions

Beat the eggs with a pinch of salt and pepper, and the oregano.

Preheat a small pan over medium heat, and melt in the butter

Pour in the eggs, and stir constantly for 3 minutes, until cooked through

Add in the feta, and stir for another minute.

Nutrition: 404 calories, 37.8 g fat, 15.3 g protein, 1.9 g net carbs

Smoked Salmon and Goat Cheese Eggs

This is an elegant, low car, high flavour breakfast! Enjoy with a few slices of cucumber or your favourite low carb bread!

Serving: 1

Serving Size: whole recipe

Prep Time: 5 minutes

Cook Time: >5 minutes

Ingredients

2 eggs, beaten

1 oz butter

1 oz goat cheese

2 oz smoked salmon

Instructions

Beat the eggs with a pinch of salt and pepper

Preheat a small pan over medium heat, and melt in the butter

Pour in the eggs, and stir constantly for 3 minutes, until cooked through

Add in the goat cheese, and stir for another minute.

Slice the salmon into thin strips, and toss with the eggs at the last minute. Serve immediately

Nutrition: 524 calories, 44.3 g fat, 30.3 g protein, 1.2 g net carbs

Dairy Free Keto Pumpkin Spice Latte

Is there anything more satisfying than a PSL? Only the satisfaction of knowing this one is ketogenic!

Serving: 1

Serving Size: whole recipe

Prep Time: >5 minutes

Cook Time: 0 minutes

Ingredients

2 eggs

1 tbsp coconut oil

1 cup hot coffee or boiling water

1 tsp pumpkin pie spice

1 tsp stevia or erythritol (optional)

Instructions

Blend the eggs, coconut oil and pumpkin spice (and sweetener, if using) in a blender for 20 seconds, to mix

Add the coffee, and blend for another minute or so

Serve immediately

Nutrition: 190 calories, 18 g fat, 6 g protein, 0.9 g net carbs

Dairy Free Keto Vanilla Latte

This vanilla latte is so easy to make, and the perfect start to your morning!

Serving: 1

Serving Size: whole recipe

Prep Time: >5 minutes

Cook Time: 0 minutes

Ingredients

2 eggs

1 tbsp coconut oil

1 cup hot coffee or boiling water

1 tsp vanilla extract

1 tsp stevia or erythritol (optional)

Instructions

Blend the eggs, coconut oil and vanilla (and sweetener, if using) in a blender for 20 seconds, to mix

Add the coffee, and blend for another minute or so

Serve immediately

Nutrition: 190 calories, 18 g fat, 6 g protein, 0.9 g net carbs

Dairy Free Keto Mocha Latte

If you're not a fan of coffee with your hot chocolate, use boiling water instead. Add a bit of cream for extra richness, if you like.

Serving: 1

Serving Size: whole recipe

Prep Time: >5 minutes

Cook Time: 0 minutes

Ingredients

2 eggs

1 tbsp coconut oil

1 cup hot coffee or boiling water

¼ tsp vanilla extract

1 tbsp cocoa powder

1 tsp stevia or erythritol (optional)

Instructions

Blend the eggs, coconut oil, vanilla, and cocoa (and sweetener, if using) in a blender for 20 seconds, to mix

Add the coffee, and blend for another minute or so

Serve immediately

Nutrition: 190 calories, 18 g fat, 6 g protein, 0.9 g net carbs

Chocolate Almond Smoothie

This caffeine free drink is full of great fat, and makes a great breakfast or snack!

Serving: 1

Serving Size: whole recipe

Prep Time: >5 minutes

Cook Time: 0 minutes

Ingredients

½ cup almond milk

1 tbsp coconut oil

2 tbsp almond butter

2 tbsp cocoa powder

1 tsp stevia or erythritol (optional)

Instructions

Blend all ingredients until smooth. Serve immediately

Nutrition: 370 calories, 33 g fat, 8 g protein, 5 g net carbs

Coconut Raspberry Smoothie

This caffeine free drink is full of great fat, and makes a great breakfast or snack!

Serving: 1

Serving Size: whole recipe

Prep Time: >5 minutes

Cook Time: 0 minutes

Ingredients

½ cup coconut milk

1 tbsp coconut oil

¼ cup frozen raspberries

1 tsp stevia or erythritol (optional)

Instructions

Blend all ingredients until smooth. Serve immediately

Nutrition: 408 calories, 42.3 g fat, 3 g protein, 6 g net carbs

Coconut Smoothie

This caffeine free drink is full of great fat, and makes a great breakfast or snack!

Serving: 1

Serving Size: whole recipe

Prep Time: >5 minutes

Cook Time: 0 minutes

Ingredients

½ cup coconut milk

1 tbsp coconut oil

½ cup ice

¼ tsp vanilla extract

1 tsp stevia or erythritol (optional)

Instructions

Blend all ingredients until smooth. Serve immediately

Nutrition: 408 calories, 42.9 g fat, 5 g protein, 3.7 g net carbs

Western Scrambled Eggs

Ham, cheese and tomato with eggs- the perfect start to your day!

Serving: 1

Serving Size: whole recipe

Prep Time: 5 minutes

Cook Time: >5 minutes

Ingredients

2 eggs, beaten

1 tsp dried thyme

1 oz butter

1 oz shredded cheddar cheese

1 oz ham, cubed

½ tomato, diced

1 tbsp red onion, diced (optional)

Instructions

Beat the eggs with a pinch of salt and pepper, and the thyme.

Preheat a small pan over medium heat, and melt in the butter

Add in the ham and tomato (and onion, if using), sauteing for 1 minute or so

Pour in the eggs, and stir constantly for 3 minutes, until cooked through

Add in the cheese, and stir for another minute.

Nutrition: 498 calories, 43.8 g fat, 23.4 g protein, 2.9 g net carbs

Mushroom, spinach and goat cheese frittata

This frittata is loaded with greens and good fat! This recipe serves two; enjoy this frittata for lunch the next day if you like- it's great hot or cold!

Serving: 2

Serving Size: Half recipe

Prep Time: 5 minutes

Cook Time: 15 minutes

Ingredients

4 eggs, beaten

¼ cup cream

1 tsp dried thyme

1 oz butter

1 oz goat cheese

1 handful spinach

½ cup sliced mushrooms

Instructions

Preheat oven to 350F

Beat the eggs and cream with a pinch of salt and pepper, and the thyme.

Preheat a small pan over medium heat, and melt in the butter

Add in the spinach and mushrooms with a pinch of salt, sauteing for 1 minute or so. Remove pan from heat.

Pour in the eggs, and top with the cheese. Transfer the pan to the oven, and bake 10-12 minutes. Store Leftovers in the fridge for up to 4 days.

Nutrition: 316 calories, 27 g fat, 16.4 g protein, 2.4 g net carbs

Bacon, Egg and Avo Breakfast Sandwich ✓

This sandwich uses two halves of an avocado for the bun- adding a ton of great fat! This is a high calorie meal, so intermittent fasting will be important later in the day.

Serving: 1

Serving Size: whole recipe

Prep Time: 5 minutes

Cook Time: 15 minutes

Ingredients

1 egg

1 oz butter

1 avocado, sliced in half

1 tsp sesame seeds (for garnish)

2 slices bacon, cooked

1 slice tomato (optional, but delicious)

1 small handful arugula or 1 leaf of romaine

Instructions

Preheat a small pan over medium heat.

Melt in the butter, and crack in the egg. Cook to desired doneness.

Lay the lettuce, tomato (if using), and bacon onto one half of the avocado. Top with the egg, and close the sandwich. Sprinkle the top half of avocado with the sesame seeds, and enjoy immediately.

Nutrition: 899 calories, 83.9 g fat, 24.2 g protein, 4.1 g net carbs

Double Egg Breakfast Sandwich

This sandwich uses two fried eggs instead of bread- giving you ALL of the good stuff, NONE of the carbs!

Serving: 1

Serving Size: whole recipe

Prep Time: 5 minutes

Cook Time: >10 minutes

Ingredients

2 eggs

1 oz butter, room temperature

1 oz ham or 2 slices bacon, cooked

2 oz shredded cheddar cheese

1 slice tomato

Instructions

Preheat oven to 350F

Grease a 2 sections of a cupcake tin with the butter, and crack an egg into each one (Prep tip- if you want to make this sandwich all week, or want eggs available pre-cooked for the week, fill all 12 slots! Cooked eggs will last for a week in the fridge!)

Bake for 5-7 minutes, until the eggs are firm. Carefully pop the eggs out of the moulds, and lay them onto a plate.

Lay the cheese on top of the first egg, then top with the ham and tomato. Close with the second egg. Serve immediately.

Nutrition: 607 calories, 53 g fat, 30.2 g protein, 2.4 g net carbs

Coconut Chia Pudding

This creamy chia pudding is so easy to prep, and really delicious!

Serving: 2

Serving Size: Half recipe

Prep Time: 5 minutes

Cook Time: >5 minutes

Ingredients

1 oz chia seeds

1 cup coconut milk

3 tbsp unsweetened coconut flakes

¼ tsp cinnamon

Instructions

Mix all ingredients together and pour into two small mason jars or sealed containers

Allow to sit in the fridge overnight

Will keep in the fridge for up to 1 week

Nutrition: 451 calories, 42 g fat, 6.6 g protein, 8 g net carbs

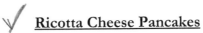 **Ricotta Cheese Pancakes**

These pancakes are the best way to start a day! Add blueberries, strawberries, or coconut for a fun twist! These pancakes can also be made with cottage cheese, goat cheese or cream cheese, if you prefer to switch it up!

Serving: 1

Serving Size: 2-3 pancakes

Prep Time: 5 minutes

Cook Time: >10 minutes

Ingredients

1 egg

2 oz Ricotta

¼ tbsp psyllium husk flour

½ oz coconut oil

1 tbsp erythritol, optional

Instructions

Beat together all ingredients, and allow to sit for a minute to thicken

Preheat a small pan over medium high heat, and melt in the coconut oil

Spoon in a dollop of pancake batter, and cook 1-2 minutes per side.

Continue until all the batter has been used up. Serve warm

Nutrition: 425 calories, 39 g fat, 14 g protein, 5 g net carbs

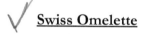 **Swiss Omelette**

Gooey cheese and ham make this omelette a delicious way to start any day!

Serving: 1

Serving Size: whole recipe

Prep Time: 5 minutes

Cook Time: 5 minutes

Ingredients

2 eggs

3 tbsp heavy cream

2 tbsp butter

1 oz ham, cubed or cut into ribbons

2 oz swiss cheese

Instructions

Beat together the eggs and cream with salt and pepper

Preheat a pan over medium heat and melt in the butter

Add in the egg mixture, and allow to cook for 3 minutes.

Flip, and cook for another minute. Lay the cheese and ham onto the top of the omelette, and carefully fold it over so that the good stuff is tucked inside. Cover the pan, and cook for 1 more minute

Nutrition: 425 calories, 39 g fat, 14 g protein, 5 g net carbs

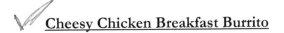 ### Cheesy Chicken Breakfast Burrito

This recipe uses leftover Lemon and Thyme Chicken Legs with cheese, Low Carb Tortillas, salsa and eggs! What a great way to start a morning!

Serving: 1

Serving Size: whole recipe

Prep Time: 10 minutes

Cook Time: 5 minutes

Ingredients

1 egg, beaten

 2 tbsp salsa

1 oz butter

1 oz shredded cheddar cheese

 1 serving Keto Tortilla

1 Serving Lemon and Thyme Chicken, shredded

Instructions

Beat the eggs and salsa together with a pinch of salt and pepper.

Preheat a small pan over medium heat, and melt in the butter

Pour in the eggs, and stir constantly for 3 minutes, until cooked through

Lay the chicken onto the tortilla, and spoon the eggs over top.

Top with the cheese, and fold the burrito. Serve immediately.

Nutrition: 830 calories, 75.2 g fat, 50.3 g protein, 3.5 g net carbs

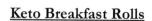

Keto Breakfast Rolls

Sometimes, you just want a soft piece of bread to start your day off right. These rolls are beautifully fluffy, and low carb! Toast them and spread some butter or nut butter for a convenient breakfast on the go, or fill them with your favourite breakfast foods to make a delicious sandwich! These can also be formed into bagels if you like.

Serving: 4

Serving Size: 1 bun

Prep Time: 15 minutes

Cook Time: 16 minutes

Ingredients

½ cup almond flour

½ cup psyllium husk fiber

1 ½ tsp xantham gum

1 egg, beaten

3 tbsp cream cheese

1 ½ cups mozzarella, shredded

1 oz butter, melted

Instructions

Preheat oven to 375F

Melt together the cream cheese and mozzarella in the microwave for 1 minute.

Meanwhile mix together the almond flour, psyllium husk and xantham gum, and beat in the egg.

Mix in the melted cheeses, stirring well until a dough has formed.

Form the dough into 4 balls, and lay onto a baking sheet lined with parchment

Brush the dough balls with the melted butter, and bake in the oven for 15 minutes.

Store leftover buns in an airtight container in the fridge for up to a week, and reheat in a 350F oven for 2-3 minutes.

Nutrition: 489 calories, 50 g fat, 30 g protein, 5.5 g net carbs

With 1 tbsp almond butter: 98 calories, 9 g fat, 3.4 g protein, 1.4 g net carbs

With 1 egg (cooked how you like): 63 calories, 4.4 g fat, 5.5 g protein, 0.3 g net carbs

<u>Smoked salmon, cream cheese and greens breakfast sandwiches</u>

These breakfast sandwiches are a great way to start the day! Use whatever greens you have on hand or like best- kale, romaine, spinach or arugula are all great options. Feel free to add a slice of tomato for a little added nutritional value.

Serving: 1

Serving Size: whole recipe

Prep Time: 10 minutes

Cook Time: 2 minutes

Ingredients

1 serving Breakfast Rolls

1/2 tbsp cream cheese

1 oz smoked salmon

Small handful greens

Instructions

Slice the breakfast roll in half, and toast for 2 minutes or so

Spread the cream cheese over the breakfast roll, and layer on the greens and salmon. Close the sandwich, and serve immediately.

Nutrition: 539 calories, 53 g fat, 35.6 g protein, 5.7 g net carbs

Coconut Matcha Latte

This latte is easy to prepare, and so so yummy! For an iced latte, just blend with ice! Because of the low caffeine content, this is a great option for the late afternoon or evening as a snack, if you're trying to watch your caffeine intake!

Serving: 1

Serving Size: whole recipe

Prep Time: 10 minutes

Cook Time: 0 minutes

Ingredients

½ tbsp erythritol

1 tbsp matcha powder

4 oz coconut milk

½ cup boiling water

Instructions

Mix all ingredients together until smooth. Serve hot, or chill for an iced latte.

Nutrition: 255 calories, 28.8 g fat, 3.4 g protein, 3 g net carbs

Halloumi Shakshouka

Shakshouka is a middle eastern dish consisting of eggs, herbs and a richly flavoured tomato sauce. We've added halloumi for an added hit of flavour and good fat.

Serving: 1

Serving Size: whole recipe

Prep Time: 5 minutes

Cook Time: >10 minutes

Ingredients

1 egg

1 tbsp tomato paste

1 tsp dried oregano

3 tbsp beef or chicken broth

1 tbsp butter

1 oz halloumi, cubed

1 tbsp fresh parsley

Instructions

Preheat oven to 350F

Grease a small ramekin (small enough to comfortably hold the egg) with the butter

Mix together the broth, tomato paste and oregano. Spoon half the mixture into the ramekin, and then crack in the egg. Top with the remaining tomato mixture

Layer the halloumi cubes gently around the egg, making sure not to crack the yolk

Bake for 5-10 minutes, until the egg white is set and the yolk is still runny. Top with parsley and serve warm.

Nutrition: 160 calories, 11.8 g fat, 3.2 g protein,1.2 g net carbs

 Cinnamon Roll Donuts

You can have donuts on the keto diet! Try these beautiful pastries with a coffee, or with a keto latte!

Serving: 6

Serving Size: 1 donut

Prep Time: 10 minutes

Cook Time: 15 minutes

Ingredients

½ cup erythritol

2 eggs

½ cup almond milk

¾ cup almond flour

½ cup psyllium husk fiber

1 tbsp cinnamon

1 tbsp baking powder

2 tbsp butter, melted

Instructions

Preheat oven to 350F

Mix together the eggs, almond milk, cinnamon, baking powder, erythritol, almond flour and psyllium husk.

Stir in the melted butter.

Grease a donut pan with a bit of butter or cooking spray, and pour the batter into the pan.

Bake for 18-20 minutes, until the donuts are set in the center. Allow to cool for 5-10 minutes, then turn out of the pan. Store leftovers in an airtight container in the fridge for up to 5 days, or freeze for up to 3 months. Reheat in the microwave for 1-2 minutes.

Nutrition: 160 calories, 11.8 g fat, 3.2 g protein,1.2 g net carbs

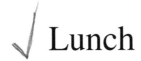 # Lunch

Green Goddess Avo Salad

This salad is so fast and easy! The avocado dressing is only good for a day, so just make what you need at the time! This is a high calorie meal! Make sure that you fast at some point today!

Serving: 1

Serving Size: whole recipe

Prep Time: 10 minutes

Cook Time: 0 Minutes

Ingredients

2 strips bacon, cooked and chopped into bits

2 cherry tomatoes, halved

½ cup romaine, chopped

1 egg, hardboiled

1 tbsp pumpkin seeds

For the dressing:

2 tbsp olive oil

½ avocado, mashed

1 tbsp white wine vinegar

1 tsp onion powder

Instructions

Make the dressing- In a blender, puree all ingredients until smooth. Adjust the consistency with a bit more oil if needed, and season with salt and pepper

Toss the dressing with the rest of the ingredients. Serve immediately, or keep in the fridge for up to 24 hours.

Nutrition: 905 calories, 75.5 g fat, 32 g protein, 10 g net carbs

Salmon, spinach and goat cheese Salad

This salad is a deliciously simple way to get a ton of nutrients and vital fats during a busy weekday

Serving: 1

Serving Size: whole recipe

Prep Time: 10 minutes

Cook Time: 0 Minutes

Ingredients

2 oz smoked salmon

½ cup spinach

1 oz goat cheese

3 cherry tomatoes, halved

1 tbsp pumpkin seeds

Instructions

Toss all ingredients together. If you wish, drizzle with a bit of avocado oil and a pinch of salt and pepper. Serve immediately.

Nutrition: 311 calories, 17.5 g fat, 24 g protein, 11 g net carbs

Beef and avocado lettuce wraps

These lettuce wraps are absolutely delicious, and so easy to make! To save time, prep your beef up to 3 days in advance!

Serving: 1

Serving Size: 4 bundles

Prep Time: 10 minutes

Cook Time: 10 Minutes

Ingredients

2 oz beef, sliced thinly

1 tbsp soy sauce (gluten free)

¼ tsp ginger

1 red chili, chopped finely

1 tbsp avocado oil

For the wraps:

4 romaine leaves

½ avocado, diced

¼ red onion, sliced

Instructions

Marinate the beef in the soy sauce, ginger, and chilis for at least 5 minutes.

Preheat a pan over medium high heat. Drizzle in the oil, and add the beef and marinade. Toss constantly for 5-10 minutes, until the beef has cooked through. Allow to cool. Store cooked beef in the fridge for up to 3 days.

Make the wraps- Lay the lettuce leaves out, and spoon in the beef, avocado and red onion. Roll up, and enjoy immediately.

Nutrition: 454 calories, 37 g fat, 21 g protein, 6 g net carbs

Keto Quesadillas

These quesadillas use Keto Tortillas for a quick, satisfying keto-friendly lunch. This is a basic quesadilla recipe (tortilla and cheese), although you can certainly make it your own by adding any of your favourite ingredients (taco meat, chicken, bacon, jalapenos, smoked salmon and cream cheese- the possibilities are endless!)

Serving: 1

Serving Size: whole recipe

Prep Time: 10 minutes

Cook Time: 6 Minutes

Ingredients

2 servings Keto Quesadillas (found in dinner recipes)

3 oz cheddar cheese

For serving:

Sour cream

Salsa

Instructions

Preheat oven to 375F

Lay one tortilla onto a baking sheet lined with parchment. Cover with cheese (and any other fillings you like), and top with the second tortilla. Bake in the oven for 6 minutes, until the cheese melts and the tortillas are golden. Slice into 4 equal pieces, and serve immediately.

Nutrition: 330 calories, 21.5 g fat, 29.7 g protein, 4.1 g net carbs

With 3 tbsp sour cream: 77 calories, 7.6 g fat, 1.1 g protein, 1.5 g carbs

Italian Chopped Salad

This salad is so big and full of all sorts of great ingredients! You'll want to eat it everyday!

Serving: 1

Serving Size: whole recipe

Prep Time: 10 minutes

Cook Time: 0 Minutes

Ingredients

3 oz mozzarella cheese, shaved or cut into chunks

3 oz proscuitto

1 egg, hardboiled

1 tomato, cut into wedges

1 cup arugula (or any other green)

6 olives

2 tbsp olive oil

1 tbsp balsamic vinegar

Handful basil

Instructions

Toss all ingredients together. Serve immediately.

Nutrition: 790 calories, 66 g fat, 47 g protein, 5.9 g net carbs

Keto Creamy Onion Poppyseed Dressing

The problem with store bought salad dressings is that they're often loaded with sugar and other preservatives. Making your own ensures that you can control exactly what's going into it. Make a batch and keep it in the fridge for whenever you need a delicious dressing or dip

Serving: 8

Serving Size: 2-3 tbsp

Prep Time: 10 minutes

Cook Time: 0 Minutes

Ingredients

¼ onion, diced

1 tsp garlic powder

1 tbsp dijon mustard

1 cup olive oil

3 tbsp poppy seeds

Instructions

In a blender, or using an immersion blender, puree together all ingredients except the poppy seeds. Mix in the seeds, and season with salt and pepper. Store in an airtight container in the fridge for up to 2 weeks.

Nutrition: 237 calories, 26.8 g fat, 1 g protein, 1 g net carbs

With ½ cup greens (spinach, arugula, or romaine) and 2 strips bacon, crumbled: 209 calories, 15.9 g fat, 14.5 g protein, 0.7 g net carbs

Keto Strawberry Balsamic Dressing

The problem with store bought salad dressings is that they're often loaded with sugar and other preservatives. This dressing is slightly sweet, slightly tangy, and goes really well with spinach and goat cheese.

Serving: 8

Serving Size: 2-3 tbsp

Prep Time: 10 minutes

Cook Time: 0 Minutes

Ingredients

2 large strawberries (frozen is fine)

2 tbsp balsamic vinegar

1 tsp dried basil

½ tbsp dijon

1 cup olive oil

Instructions

Blend together all ingredients until smooth and creamy. Season with salt and pepper.

Nutrition: 220 calories, 25.2 g fat, 0 g protein, 0.3 g net carbs

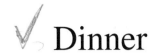 # Dinner

Warm mushrooms and brown butter

Serve this mushroom side with your favourite protein (it goes amazingly well with red meat, but is also delicious with fish or chicken!). Any leftovers are delicious on top of spinach for a healthy salad the next day

Serving: 2

Serving Size: Half recipe

Prep Time: 5 minutes

Cook Time: >10 Minutes

Ingredients

3 cups mushrooms, sliced

3 oz butter

2 tbsp dried thyme

3 tsp garlic powder

1 tsp onion powder

3 tbsp heavy cream

Instructions

Preheat a medium pan over medium high heat.

Melt in the butter, and add in the thyme, garlic, and onion powder. Reduce the heat to medium low, and cook the butter until it foams and begins to darken in colour, about 3 minutes.

Add the mushrooms with a pinch of salt, and saute well for 5 minutes until they have begun to cook down.

Serve over your favourite protein. Refrigerate any leftovers in an airtight container for up to 4 days- this is delicious hot or cold!

Nutrition: 500 calories, 47 g fat, 18 g protein, 6 g net carbs

Plus 4 oz steak: 226 cal, 5.7 g fat, 41 g protein, 0 g carbs

Plus salmon: 150 cal, 7 g fat, 22 g protein, 0 g carbs

Asian Style Beef Salad

This salad is packed with flavour and really delicious! It makes an awesome dinner, and an even better lunch the next day!

Serving: 2

Serving Size: Half recipe

Prep Time: 15 minutes

Cook Time: 10 Minutes

Ingredients

For the Beef:

1 tbsp sesame oil

1 tbsp fish sauce

1 tbsp ginger

2 tsp chili flakes (or as much or as little as you like)

1 tsp tamari

1 lb steak (such as flank steak or rib eye), thinly sliced

For the sesame aioli:

1 tbsp mayo

1 tsp sesame oil

1 tsp avocado oil

½ lime, juice and zest

For the salad:

3 cherry tomatoes, halved

½ cucumber, spiralized or cut into thin strips

1 carrot, spiralized or cut into thin strips

1 cup iceberg lettuce, finely chopped

3 green onions, sliced

Handful fresh cilantro

Instructions

Cook the beef- Toss the beef with the rest of the ingredients, and allow to marinate for 5-10 minutes

 Preheat a medium pan over medium high heat.

Add the beef with the marinade, and toss well for 10 minutes, until fully cooked.

Make the aioli- Mix all ingredients together until smooth.

Make the salad- Toss together all ingredients. Toss in the warm beef. Drizzle with the aioli, and toss once more to combine.

Nutrition: 603 calories, 22 g fat, 85.2 g protein, 5 g net carbs

 Cauliflower and goat cheese mash

This pureed cauliflower is the perfect substitute for mashed potatoes! In this recipe, the cauliflower is enhanced with creamy goat cheese and roasted garlic, but you can easily keep this simple with just cream and butter, or mix in some bacon and cheddar cheese for a delicious comfort food experience. Serve this decadent side with a piece of protein (steak, chicken or fish all work great with this) and a serving of greens for a complete meal that will please everyone!

Serving: 4

Serving Size: Half recipe

Prep Time: 5 minutes

Cook Time: 40 Minutes

Ingredients

1 head cauliflower, chopped

1 cup heavy cream

6 oz goat cheese

4 oz butter

1 head garlic

¼ cup olive oil

Instructions

Preheat oven to 400F. Lay the head of garlic in a small, oven safe container.

Slice the top off the head of garlic (leaving the cloves intact), and pour the oil all over it. Sprinkle with a pinch of salt. Roast 15 minutes, until fragrant and soft, then allow to cool while you move on to the next step.

In a large pot, bring 4 cups of water to a boil. Boil the cauliflower for 5 minutes, until soft. Drain, and set aside.

Preheat a large sized sauce pan over medium heat. Pop the roasted garlic cloves out of their skin, and add it to the pan with the butter. Stir constantly until the butter has melted completely, then add in the cream and the cauliflower, continuing to stir for 5 minutes.

Using an immersion blender or food processor, puree the cauliflower until completely smooth.

Continue to cook over medium heat for another 10 minutes, until the mixture has thickened. Stir in the goat cheese, and season with salt and pepper. Keep leftovers in an airtight container in the fridge for up to 7 days.

Nutrition: 559 calories, 54.1 g fat, 15 g protein, 4.6 g net carbs

Plus 4 oz steak: 226 cal, 5.7 g fat, 41 g protein, 0 g carbs

Plus 4 oz salmon: 150 cal, 7 g fat, 22 g protein, 0 g carbs

Plus 1 roasted chicken leg, skin on: 553 cal, 15.7 g fat, 30.5 g protein, 0 carbs

Plus 1 chicken breast, skin on: 193 cal, 7.6 g fat, 29.2 g protein, 0 carbs

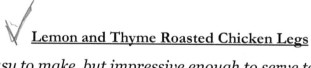

Lemon and Thyme Roasted Chicken Legs

This chicken dish so easy to make, but impressive enough to serve to guests! The juicy, high fat dark meat is perfect for the ketogenic diet, so enjoy these as often as you like! If you're a fan of breasts, this method will work great for that too! Chicken legs are considered the thigh and drum attached.

Serving: 4

Serving Size: 1 leg

Prep Time: 5 minutes

Cook Time: 45 Minutes

Ingredients

4 large chicken legs, bone in skin on

1 bunch fresh thyme, chopped

2 cloves garlic, minced

¼ cup butter, softened

1 lemon, zested and cut into wheels

Instructions

Preheat oven to 350F. Prepare a roasting pan by laying down the lemon wheels, then placing the chicken thighs over top.

Mix together the thyme, garlic, lemon zest and butter.

Lift the skin slightly from the meat of the chicken, and stuff the butter mixture under the skin. Continue until all 4 chicken thighs are done

Season the top of the skin with salt and pepper, then bake the chicken for 35-40 minutes, until completely cooked through. Serve with your favourite sides. Leftovers will keep in the fridge for up to 4 days.

Nutrition: 379 calories, 27.8 g fat, 30.5 g protein, 0.6 g net carbs

Bacon Wrapped Cod

This recipe is really easy and delicious! Serve with your favourite sides for a complete, beautiful meal.

Serving: 2

Serving Size: 1 fillet

Prep Time: 5 minutes

Cook Time: 20 Minutes

Ingredients

2 4 oz fillets cod

4 strips bacon

Instructions

Preheat oven to 350F

Pat the cod dry, and season with salt and pepper. Wrap two slices of bacon around each fillet, and lay them onto a baking sheet lined with parchment.

Bake 20 minutes. Serve with your favourite sides. Leftovers will keep in the fridge for up to two days.

Nutrition: 323 calories, 27.6 g fat, 17.5 g protein, 0.7 g net carbs

Bacon-Parmesan Roasted Asparagus

This yummy side dish is the perfect addition to any meal, but also makes a great lunch or snack on its own. Asparagus gives you the greens you need, without a lot of extra carbs.

Serving: 4

Serving Size: 3 spears

Prep Time: 5 minutes

Cook Time: 22 Minutes

Ingredients

12 asparagus spears, trimmed

4 slices bacon

¼ cup olive oil

1 tsp garlic powder

½ cup parmesan, grated

Instructions

Preheat oven to 400F

Bring a large pot of salted water to a boil, and blanch the asparagus for 1 minute. Transfer to an ice bath.

Lay the asparagus out onto a baking sheet lined with parchment, and drizzle with oil. Toss together the garlic and parmesan, and sprinkle over the asparagus evenly.

Divide the stalks into bundles of 3, and wrap each bundle with a strip of bacon. Bake for 20 minutes.

 ### Creamy Bacon and Spinach Zucchini Noodles

This recipe is fast, easy, and delicious! It can be eaten on its own, but also makes a great side! Serve with your favourite protein for a complete meal. This is a high calorie item, so make sure you incorporate intermittent fasting in your day as well!

Serving: 2

Serving Size: Half of recipe

Prep Time: 15 minutes

Cook Time: 25 Minutes

Ingredients

4 strips bacon, diced

½ cup heavy cream

2 cloves garlic, minced

½ cup parmesan, grated

¼ cup olive oil

4 zucchinis, spiralized

Instructions

Preheat a large pan over medium heat. Add in the olive oil and bacon, and cook until bacon is cooked through, about 2 minutes. Add in the garlic, and saute for another minute.

Pour in the cream, and reduce heat to low. Allow to simmer for 10 minutes.

Add in the zucchini noodles, and toss well to combine. Cook for about 10 minutes until cooked through. Serve immediately or keep leftovers in a container in the fridge for up to 3 days.

Nutrition: 770 calories, 65 g fat, 37.6 g protein, 12 g net carbs

Pesto Chicken Casserole

This is such a comforting meal! If you want to switch it up, swap out chicken for sausage, pork, or anything else. If you have previously cooked chicken from another recipe, save yourself time by using that instead of raw chicken thighs!

Serving: 4

Serving Size: about 1 cup

Prep Time: 15 minutes

Cook Time: 45 Minutes

Ingredients

12 oz chicken thighs, bones removed and diced into small pieces

½ onion, diced

1 tsp dried thyme

1 tsp dried basil

1 oz butter

3 oz pesto (jarred is fine- just read the ingredients to make sure there are no added sugars!)

1 cup heavy cream

½ red pepper, diced

2 oz parmesan cheese

2 oz mozzarella cheese

Instructions

Preheat oven to 400F

Preheat a dutch oven or ovensafe pan over medium high heat, and melt in the butter. Add in the chicken with a pinch of salt and pepper, and the basil and thyme. Cook for 5-10 minutes, until all sides are browned

Mix together the pesto, cream, and diced red bell pepper

Pour the mixture in with the chicken, and top with the cheeses

Bake covered for 35-40 minutes. Serve warm with a side of greens. Leftovers will last in the fridge for up to a week.

Southwest Chicken Chili with Avocado Cream

This white chili leaves out the legumes and focuses on meat and flavour! If you have leftover cooked chicken from a previous recipe, save yourself time by using it in the recipe instead of uncooked thighs. You can swap out chicken for beef or pork if you like. The avocado cream is delicious on top of this recipe, but also makes a great topper for salads, or an alternative to mayo!

Serving: 4

Serving Size: about 1 cup

Prep Time: 5 minutes

Cook Time: 40 Minutes

Ingredients

½ lb chicken thighs, skinless, boneless and diced

½ lb chicken breasts, skinless, boneless and diced

2 tbsp olive or avocado oil

1 onion, diced

3 cloves garlic, minced

1 tbsp cumin

2 tbsp chili powder

1 tsp cinnamon

½ tbsp dried oregano

2 jalapenos, diced (optional)

1 bell pepper, diced

1 8 oz can diced tomatoes

1 cup chicken stock

Handful cilantro, for garnish

For the avocado cream:

1 avocado, mashed

¼ cup heavy cream

Instructions

Preheat a large pot over medium high heat.

Drizzle in the oil, and add in the chicken, spices, salt and pepper. Brown the chicken on all sides (about 10 minutes), then remove from the pan.

Add in another drizzle of oil, and toss in the peppers, onion and garlic. Stir well for 3-5 minutes. Add the chicken back in, along with the diced tomatoes and stock. Bring to a boil, then reduce heat to low. Let simmer for 20-25 minutes, stirring occasionally.

Make the avocado cream- mash the avocado well, and combine with the cream in a small bowl. Beat with a whisk until smooth. Taste, and season with salt and pepper.

To serve, pour the chili into a bowl and top with a bit of cilantro (optional) and a big scoop of avocado cream. Serve immediately. Leftover chili will keep in the fridge for up to a week, avocado cream will keep in the fridge for 1 day.

Nutrition: 410 calories 23.1 g fat, 28.9 g protein, 7 g net carbs

Roulade of chicken with ricotta, spinach and lemon cream

This might sound fancy, but it's super easy to put together! Impress your guests, or just enjoy this all by yourself on a weeknight! Serve with a side of asparagus, or a green salad. You can also swap out the ricotta for goat cheese or cream cheese, if you prefer. This is a high calorie meal, so make sure you incorporate fasting in your day.

Serving: 2

Serving Size: 1 breast

Prep Time: 10 minutes

Cook Time: 30 Minutes

Ingredients

2 6 oz boneless skinless chicken breasts

1 cup spinach

1 oz ricotta cheese

1 tbsp butter, softened

1 tbsp olive oil

1 tbsp thyme

For the cream:

½ cup heavy cream

1 oz parmesan

1 lemon, zest only

Instructions

Preheat oven to 350F

Cut an incision through the center of the breast (making sure not to go all the way through!), and then run your knife under each side so that the breast opens like a book

In a small bowl, mix together the butter, ricotta, and spinach, and season with a pinch of salt and pepper

Spoon the filling into the center of each chicken breast, and fold the sides back up to close

Brush the chicken with the olive oil, and sprinkle on the thyme, as well as some salt and pepper. Bake for 30 minutes

While the chicken is baking, add the cream and lemon zest to a small saucepan and warm it over medium heat, stirring constantly for 3-5 minutes.

Reduce the heat to low, and cook for another 15 minutes, stirring occasionally. Stir in the cheese and keep warm until ready to serve.

To serve, slice the chicken breasts into 3 or 4 equal sized medallions. Spoon the sauce over top. Serve warm or cold. Leftovers will keep in the fridge for up to a week

Nutrition: 700 calories 63.8 g fat, 72.9 g protein, 3.6 g net carbs

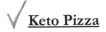 **Keto Pizza**

Pizza nights can still happen on the keto diet! This crust is made with cheese instead of flour, making it deliciously decadent and keto friendly! This is a basic recipe for pepperoni pizza, but you can also add whichever toppings you like- as long as they're keto friendly, and you make sure to take the extra macros into consideration.

Serving: 2

Serving Size: Half Pizza

Prep Time: 10 minutes

Cook Time: 30 Minutes

Ingredients

For the crust:

4 oz mozzarella

4 oz parmesan

6 eggs

For the topping:

4 oz mozzarella, shredded

¼ cup Low carb tomato sauce (check the label, make sure it's sugar free)

1 oz Pepperoni

Instructions

Preheat oven to 425F

Make the crust- In a bowl, mix together the parm, mozzarella, and eggs. Lay the mixture out onto a baking sheet or pizza stone lined with parchment, flattening it into a large circle- for personal size pizzas, just make two equal sized circles

Bake for 10 minutes, until the cheese has melted and it resembles a crust. Carefully remove the crust from the oven, making sure not to disturb it. Let it cool for at least 5-10 minutes

Spread the sauce and toppings on top of the crust, and return to the oven for another 10 minutes. Allow to cool for 5 minutes before slicing. Leftovers will last in the fridge for up to a week.

Nutrition: 761 calories 52 g fat, 70 g protein, 7 g net carbs

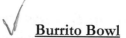 **Burrito Bowl**

Everybody knows the best part of a burrito bowl is the meat and cheese anyway, so leave those beans and rice out and replace them with MORE of the good stuff! If you really need rice, cauliflower rice is a great addition to this meal. If you have leftover beef from Taco night, feel free to use it in this recipe!

Serving: 2

Serving Size: Half recipe

Prep Time: 10 minutes

Cook Time: 30 Minutes

Ingredients

1/2 lb ground beef

1 tbsp onion powder

1 tbsp garlic powder

1 tsp cayenne (or as much as you like)

½ tbsp cumin

½ tbsp oregano

3 oz shredded cheddar cheese

6 green onions, sliced

Handful cilantro, chopped

½ bell pepper, diced

½ avocado, sliced

Instructions

Preheat a pan over medium high heat

Add in the beef and spices with some salt, and cook until the beef has cooked through- about 10 minutes

Add in the bell pepper, and toss well.

Spoon the mixture into two bowls, and top with the cheese, green onions, cilantro and avocado. Serve with your favourite salsa if you like.

Nutrition: 545 calories 32 g fat, 48.6 g protein, 11 g net carbs

 Keto Cabbage Rolls

This Eastern European classic dinner is a surefire hit! Cabbage, loaded with ground beef and pork, and topped with a rich beefy tomato sauce, this recipe is low cal and high flavour!

Serving: 4

Serving Size: 3 rolls

Prep Time: 10 minutes

Cook Time: 1 hour 30 Minutes

Ingredients

1 lb ground beef

½ lb ground pork

1 tbsp onion powder

1 tbsp garlic powder

1 tsp cayenne (or as much as you like)

12 large cabbage leaves

1 egg

For the sauce:

1 can diced tomatoes

1 cup beef stock

½ tbsp onion powder

1 tsp worchestershire sauce

1 tsp oregano

2 tbsp butter

Instructions

Preheat oven to 350F

Make the sauce- In a large saucepan, combine all ingredients and bring to a boil. Reduce heat to low, and simmer for 15 minutes. Puree with an immersion blender, or transfer to a blender or food processor until smooth.

Bring a large pot of water to a boil

Boil the cabbage leaves for 3 minutes, until tender, then drain.

Combine the beef, pork, seasonings, and egg in a bowl. Season with salt and pepper.

Lay the cabbage leaves out evenly into a roasting pan.

Spoon the meat mixture into the center of each leaf, and roll it up.

Cover the rolls with the sauce, and cover the roasting pan. Bake for 75 minutes.

Nutrition: 405 calories, 16.4 g fat, 53.6 g protein, 7 g net carbs

Pork Chops with Mushrooms

These easy pork chops are delicious, and go great with asparagus, cauliflower puree, or a simple salad. This is a high calorie meal! Make sure you fast at some point during the day!

Serving: 2

Serving Size: 1 pork chop

Prep Time: 10 minutes

Cook Time: 45 Minutes

Ingredients

2 6 oz pork chops

1 cup mushrooms, chopped

6 stems fresh thyme, leaves removed and chopped

3 tbsp butter

3/4 cup heavy cream

1 clove garlic, minced

1 oz parmesan

Handful fresh parsley, chopped

Instructions

Preheat oven to 350F

Make the sauce- Preheat a large pan over medium heat. Melt in the butter, and add the mushrooms, garlic and thyme. Saute for 2 minutes or so, until the mushrooms begin to cook down- be careful not to burn the butter!

Add in the cream, and stir for 5 minutes. Reduce heat to low, and simmer for 20 minutes. Stir in the parmesan during the last minute of cooking.

Meanwhile, roast the pork- Pat the pork chops dry, and lay them on a baking sheet lined with parchment. Season both sides with salt and pepper, and bake for 30 minutes.

Spoon the sauce over the pork chops. Garnish with chopped parsley. Leftovers will keep in the fridge for up to a week.

Nutrition: 805 calories, 73.4 g fat, 45.6 g protein, 3.4 g net carbs

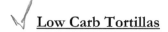 **Low Carb Tortillas**

These tortillas are perfect for tacos and wraps, and are keto friendly! Make a big batch and freeze them individually, so that you can have a low carb mexican meal any time you like!

Serving: 6

Serving Size: 1 tortilla

Prep Time: 10 minutes

Cook Time: 5 Minutes

Ingredients

3 egg whites

1 whole egg

4 oz cream cheese

1 tbsp psyllium husk fiber

1 tbsp coconut flour

Instructions

Preheat oven to 400F

Whip the egg whites until fluffy.

Beat together the cream cheese and the whole egg. Add in the flours, continuing to beat well. Fold in the egg whites.

Divide the mixture into 6 equal sized balls. Lay the balls out onto a baking sheet lined with parchment, and press them down to flatten them.

Bake for 5 minutes, until the tortilla has started to brown. Allow to cool fully before handling. Leftovers will keep in the fridge for up to two weeks, or in the freezer for 5 months.

Nutrition: 95 calories, 7.6 g fat, 4.5 g protein, 1.3 g net carbs

Keto Taco Night

These tortillas are perfect for tacos and wraps, and are keto friendly! Make a big batch and freeze them individually, so that you can have a low carb mexican meal any time you like!

Serving: 2

Serving Size: 2 tacos

Prep Time: 10 minutes

Cook Time: 45 Minutes

Ingredients

3/4 lb ground beef

2 tbsp olive or avocado oil

½ onion, diced

1 tsp garlic powder

2 tsp cumin

2 tsp chili powder

2 tsp oregano

½ tsp cinnamon

Toppings:

½ cup iceberg lettuce, shredded

½ cup cheddar cheese, shredded

Salsa

½ avocado, diced

Handful cilantro, chopped

4 servings Keto Tortillas

Instructions

Preheat a pan over medium high heat

Drizzle in the oil, and add in the onion, seasonings, and a pinch of salt. Saute until the onions become fragrant, about 5 minutes

Add in the beef. Stir well to combine, and cook completely- about 10 minutes.

To serve, spoon the filling out into the center of each taco. Top as desired, and eat immediately

Nutrition: 860 calories, 77.6 g fat, 54.5 g protein, 3.9 g net carbs

Oysters Rockefeller

This New Orleans classic has made a big comeback lately- mainly because it is ABSOLUTELY delicious! Oysters are baked with cream, butter, cheese, bacon and spinach for a high fat, high flavour seafood option.

Serving: 2

Serving Size: 6 oysters

Prep Time: 10 minutes

Cook Time: 25 Minutes

Ingredients

4 strips bacon, diced

1 tbsp butter

½ cup heavy cream

½ cup spinach

1 jalapeno, diced

1 clove garlic, minced

1 tsp thyme

12 oysters, shucked

2 oz parmesan, shredded

2 oz mozzarella, shredded

Instructions

Preheat broiler to 550F

Preheat a pan over medium heat. Melt in the butter, and cook the bacon until just cooked, about 2 minutes. Add in the thyme, garlic, and cook for another 2 minutes or so.

Add the cream and the jalapeno, and stir well for 3 minutes. Add in the spinach, tossing well to combine. Cook on medium until the spinach has cooked down and the liquid has reduced down a bit, about 6 minutes

Spoon the mixture into the oysters, and top with the cheese. Broil for 10 minutes, until the cheese is bubbling. Serve immediately.

Nutrition: 700 calories, 55.6 g fat, 60.9 g protein, 13 g net carbs

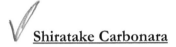

Shiratake Carbonara

Shiratake noodles are a miraculously delicious low carb noodle! This creamy carbonara recipe is easy to make, and delicious

Serving: 2

Serving Size: Half recipe

Prep Time: 10 minutes

Cook Time: 15 Minutes

Ingredients

12 strips bacon, diced

2 tbsp butter

1 tsp thyme

1 tbsp diced onion

¼ onion, diced

1 egg yolk

1 cup heavy cream

2 oz parmesan cheese

1 8 oz package shiratake noodles

Instructions

Preheat a pan over medium heat. Melt in the butter, and cook the bacon until just cooked, about 2 minutes. Add in the thyme, onion and garlic, and cook for another 2 minutes or so.

Add the cream and stir well for 1 minute. Whisk in the egg yolks one at a time, mixing well between each addition.

Add in the noodles, and toss well to combine. Allow to cook for 3-5 minutes, until the noodles have absorbed the sauce. Toss in the cheese, and season with salt and pepper. Leftovers will keep in the fridge for up to a week.

Nutrition: 720 calories, 67 g fat, 33.9 g protein, 4.7 g net carbs

Coconut Curry Shiratake Noodles

These noodles are creamy, spicy and really yummy!

Serving: 2

Serving Size: Half recipe

Prep Time: 10 minutes

Cook Time: 15 Minutes

Ingredients

1 tbsp avocado oil

6 oz chicken thighs, boneless, skinless, diced

1 8 oz can coconut milk

1 tbsp curry powder

2 red chilies (or as many as you like)

1 tsp ginger

1 clove garlic, minced

1 8 oz package bean sprouts

Handful cilantro

1 lime, juice and zest

½ bell pepper, sliced thinly

6 green onions, sliced thinly

1 8 oz package shiratake noodles

Instructions

Preheat a large pan over medium heat. Drizzle in the oil, and add the chicken with a pinch of salt. Cook until brown on all sides, about 5 minutes.

Add in the garlic, ginger, chilies, and curry powder, and stir well. Add in the coconut milk, and bring to a boil, then reduce heat to low and simmer for 10 minutes until the mixture has thickened

Add in the shiratake noodles, tossing well to combine. Add in the bell pepper and bean sprouts. Toss well. Squeeze in the lime juice, and toss in the cilantro and green onions. Serve warm. Leftovers will keep in the fridge for up to a week.

Nutrition: 557 calories, 41.7 g fat, 33.7 g protein, 13 g net carbs

Middle Eastern Style Halloumi

Halloumi is a middle eastern cheese that is slightly salty and perfectly melty. Crispy cucumbers, red onion and tomatoes make this a perfectly rounded dinner.

Serving: 1

Serving Size: whole recipe

Prep Time: 10 minutes

Cook Time: 5 Minutes

Ingredients

For the halloumi:

4 oz wedge of halloumi

½ tsp cumin

¼ tsp sumac

¼ tsp coriander

¼ tsp cinnamon

¼ tsp turmeric

For the salad:

2 tbsp red onion, diced

½ cucumber, diced

1 roma tomato, diced

Handful parsley, chopped finely

1 serving Tahini

Instructions

Preheat broiler to 500F

Mix the spices together and rub them into both sides of the cheese

Lay the halloumi out onto a baking sheet lined with parchment, and broil for 3-4 minutes, until golden and soft.

Toss together the red onion, cucumber, tomato and parsley. Spoon the tahini over top. Lay the halloumi on top, and serve immediately

Nutrition: 700 calories, 53.2 g fat, 33.7 g protein, 15 g net carbs

Tahini

Tahini is a creamy, flavourful sauce that can be used on salads, sandwiches, or as a dip!

Serving: 4

Serving Size: 2-3 tbsp

Prep Time: 10 minutes

Cook Time: 0 Minutes

Ingredients

Handful parsley, roughly chopped

1 clove garlic

1 lemon, juice and zest

¼ cup tahini paste

¼ cup water

Instructions

Puree all ingredients until smooth. Season with salt.

Keep in an airtight container in the fridge for up to a week.

Nutrition: 89 calories, 8.1 g fat, 2.5 g protein, 1.3 g net carbs

Eggplant Parmesan

This delicious vegetarian keto recipe is super rich and delicious! Use the same method to make chicken parmesan too!

Serving: 4

Serving Size: 1-2 pieces eggplant

Prep Time: 10 minutes

Cook Time: 45 Minutes

Ingredients

1 large eggplant, sliced into medallions

3 tbsp olive oil

4 oz shredded mozzarella

5 oz parmesan

1 cup marinara sauce (make sure it's low carb!)

1 tbsp garlic powder

1 tbsp onion powder

1 tbsp dried thyme

1 tbsp dried oregano

Fresh parsley, chopped

Instructions

Preheat oven to 450F

Brush the eggplant medallions with oil, and season with salt, pepper and the seasonings. Lay the medallions into a roasting pan.

Top the medallions evenly with half of the parmesan, and bake for 5 minutes

Remove from the oven, and reduce the oven temp to 375

Pour the marinara sauce over the eggplant. Top with the rest of the cheese, and cover with tinfoil. Bake for 40 minutes. Finish with parsley.

Nutrition: 385 calories, 28.1 g fat, 22.5 g protein, 12.3 g net carbs

Weekly Shopping List

*Note- It can be more economical to purchase meat items in bulk. Portioning out your meat items and freezing them will save time and money later.

Pantry Staples For the Month:

Almond Milk- 6 L

Curry Powder- 1 package, about 300g

Cumin- 1 package, about 300g

Ground Ginger- 1 package, about 300g OR 1 root

Onion Powder 1 package, about 300g

Garlic Powder 1 package, about 300g

Cinnamon 1 package, about 300g

Pumpkin Pie Spice- 1 pack, about 300g

Dried Italian herbs 1 package, about 300g

Turmeric-   1 package, about 300g

Sumac-   1 package, about 300g

Coriander-   1 package, about 300g

Poppyseeds- 1 package, about 300g

Baking powder

Tahini- 1 jar

Sugar Free Sriracha Sauce- 1 bottle

Gluten Free Tamari or soy sauce - 1 bottle

Vanilla extract

Pesto- 2 jars

Salsa- 1 jar

Olives- 2 jars

Tomato Paste- 2 jars

Marinara sauce (sugar free)- 2 jars

Balsamic vinegar- 1 bottle

Fish sauce- 1 bottle

Coconut oil

Sesame oil- 1 bottle

Coffee- 1 lb

Avocado Oil

Olive Oil

Salt

Pepper

Beef Stock- either 3L prepared, or bouillon cubes

Chicken Stock- either 3L prepared, or bouillon cubes

Pecans 6 oz

Almonds 6 oz

macadamia nuts 6 oz

Chia Seeds 16 oz

Coconut flour- 8 oz

Matcha powder- 4 oz

Unsweetened coconut flakes- 1 package

Cocoa powder- 1 can

Psyllium Husk Fiber- 8 oz

Erythritol- 8 oz

Frozen strawberries- 1 bag

Week 1 Shopping List

Seafood, Meat and Eggs:

Eggs- 2 dozen

Salmon- 4 oz

Smoked Salmon- 1 lb

Bacon- 1 lb

Steak- 12 oz

Chicken Legs- 1 package (about 1 lb)

Ham- 1 package (about 6 oz)

Cod- 2x 4 oz fillets

Dairy Products:

Feta Cheese- 8 oz

Goat Cheese- 8 oz

Cheddar cheese- 1 lb

Butter- 1 lb

Heavy Cream- 1 L

Mozzarella- 6 oz

Parmesan Cheese- 12 oz

Produce:

Spinach- 1 lb

Mushrooms- 1 lb

Avocados- 4

1 eggplant

Asparagus- 1 bunch

Cauliflower- 1 head

3 lemons

1 head romaine

1 bell pepper

1 head garlic

1 package red chilies

2 roma tomatoes

1 lb carrots

1 red onion

Yellow onions- 1 lb

Celery- 1 head

Week 2 Shopping List

Meat and Eggs:

Chicken thighs- 1 lb

Chicken Legs- 1 lb

Ground beef- 1 lb

Prosciutto- 8 oz

Bacon- 1 lb

Eggs- 1 dozen

Dairy Products:

Halloumi- 1 lb

Ricotta Cheese- 8 oz

Produce:

2 roma tomatoes

1 Pint Cherry Tomatoes

3 lemons

2 Avocados

2 jalapenos

1 bell pepper

1 bunch cilantro

1 lime

1 red onion

1 bunch parsley

Kalamata olives- 1 lb

1 bunch arugula

1 bunch fresh thyme

4 zucchinis

1 head garlic

Week 3 Shopping List

Meat and Eggs:

Ground beef- 1 lb

Ham- 4 oz

Bacon- 2 lbs

Eggs- 2 dozen

Prosciutto- 8 oz

Pepperoni- 1 lb

Steak- 12 oz

Cod- 2 4 oz fillets

Chicken Breasts- 1 package (2 lbs)

Smoked salmon- 1 lb

Dairy Products:

Feta Cheese- 1 lb

Halloumi- 1 lb

Cream cheese- 16 oz

Cream- 1 L

Butter- 1 lb

goat cheese - 8 oz

Cheddar Cheese- 1 lb

Mozzarella- 1 lb

Sour cream- 8 oz

Swiss cheese- 8 oz

Produce:

Cabbage- 1 head

2 roma tomatoes

1 package cherry tomatoes

1 red onion

1 head romaine lettuce

½ lb Spinach

Mushrooms- 1 lb

Cauliflower-1 Head

1 Package Fresh Basil

Asparagus 1 bunch

1 Lime

1 Bunch Cilantro

2 lemons

2 jalapenos

1 bunch green onions

Mixed greens

Week 4 Shopping List

Meat and Eggs:

Chicken Breast-1 lb

Chicken thighs- 1 pack, about 2 lbs

Bacon 1 lb

Eggs- 1 dozen

Chicken thighs- 1 lb

Oysters- 12 individual (purchase on or before the day you plan on using them)

Prosciutto- 8 oz

Cod- 6 oz

Ham- 8 oz

Pork chops- 8 oz

Dairy Products:

Goat Cheese- 8 oz

Heavy Cream- 8 oz

Butter 1 lb

Mozzarella- 1 lb

Produce:

1 bunch Asparagus

3 Avocados

1 package spinach

1 Package Fresh Basil

1 Head Cauliflower

1 eggplant

3 zucchini

Mushrooms- 1 lb

3 Bell Peppers

1 Cucumber

1 Tomato

1 pint cherry tomatoes

4 Onions

2 lemons

1 lime

1 bunch green onions

BREAKFAST

Coconut Smoothie Bowl

Mix in your favorite nuts and seeds to add valuable fat, texture and flavor! Be mindful of how many berries you add, so that you don't consume too many carbs

Serving: 1

Serving Size: whole recipe

Prep Time: 5 minutes

Cook Time: 0 minutes

Ingredients

1 can coconut cream

1 lime, juice and zest

¼ cup fresh raspberries

¼ cup chopped almonds

2 tbsp chia seeds

1 tbsp stevia or erythritol, optional

Instructions

Mix together the coconut, lime, and stevia (if using).

Top with the almonds, raspberries and chia seeds. Serve immediately, or store in an airtight container in the fridge for up to 12 hours.

Nutrition: 726 calories, 69.4 g fat, 11.4 g protein, 6 g net carbs

Microwave Scrambled Eggs

Using the microwave, you can have delicious scrambled eggs in less than 5 minutes! Greasing your ramekin or bowl before cracking in the eggs adds a nice bit of fat and keeps the eggs from sticking. Add in your favourite ingredients, including sliced mushrooms, chopped pepper or tomato, spinach, cheese or bacon, and enjoy!

Serving: 1

Serving Size: whole recipe

Prep Time: 5 minutes

Cook Time: 3-5 minutes, depending on add-ins

Ingredients

1 tbsp butter or olive oil

3 eggs, beaten

2 tbsp heavy cream

Salt and pepper, to taste

Instructions

Grease a microwave safe bowl well with the butter or oil

Beat together the eggs, cream and seasonings. If you're adding in any extra ingredients, do so now.

Cover the bowl with a plate or a lid (make sure it's microwave safe!), and pop into the microwave.

Cook on high for 2 minutes. Give it a quick stir, and cook at 1 minute intervals until cooked through.

Nutrition: 394 calories, 35.7 g fat, 17.4 g protein, 0.1 g net carbs

Green Smoothie

Getting your greens has never been more delicious! If you have a hard time with green smoothies, try freezing the avocado and adding some crushed ice, to make a smoothie bowl instead! Top with a few berries and nuts for a touch of sweetness and texture if you desire.

Serving: 1

Serving Size: whole recipe

Prep Time: 5 minutes

Cook Time: 0 minutes

Ingredients

1 Cup of Spinach

1/2 Avocado

¼ Cup Coconut Milk

1 Tablespoon Chia Seeds

Instructions

Pour the coconut milk into a high speed blender or food processor

Add in the rest of the ingredients, and puree until smooth. Drink immediately.

Nutrition: 350 calories, 34 fat, 4.1 g protein, 1.5 g net carbs

 Chicken Parm Frittata

Use leftover Cheesy Chicken Bake to make this quick, easy frittata in a flash!

Serving: 2

Serving Size: Half of recipe

Prep Time: 1 minute

Cook Time: 12 minutes

Ingredients

1 serving Cheesy Chicken Bake (found in dinner recipes)

2 eggs, beaten

Instructions

Preheat oven to 400F

Mix together the eggs and chicken mixture in an oven safe dish or ramekin large enough to fit everything comfortably.

Bake for 12 minutes, until cooked through. Serve immediately, and store any leftovers in an airtight container for up to 7 days.

Nutrition: 600 calories, 31 g fat, 45 g protein, 9.3 g net carbs

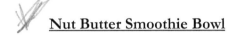 ## Nut Butter Smoothie Bowl

This nutty smoothie bowl is decadently delicious and full of good fat to fuel your morning!

Serving: 1

Serving Size: about 1 cup

Prep Time: 5 minutes

Cook Time: 0 minutes

Ingredients

2 tbsp Almond butter

1 Cup Almond milk

¼ cup ice

1 Tbsp Hemp Seeds

1 tbsp chia seeds

1 tbsp walnuts

Instructions

In a blender, puree together the ice, almond butter and almond milk until smooth.

Spoon the mixture into a bowl, and top with the hemp, walnuts and chia seeds. Serve immediately.

Nutrition: 183 calories, 13.3g fat, 8.6 g protein, 0.1 g net carbs

Blue Smoothie

This vibrant blue smoothie is just the thing to get you going in the morning! Spirulina powder is a great way to supplement your diet with a bit more green power, and also contains fiber, making it a welcome addition to this breakfast treat!

Serving: 1

Serving Size: about 1 cup

Prep Time: 5 minutes

Cook Time: 0 minutes

Ingredients

½ cup frozen blueberries

1 cup almond milk

1 tbsp coconut oil

1 tbsp spirulina

1 tsp stevia or erythritol, optional

Instructions

In a blender, puree everything together until smooth. Serve immediately.

Nutrition: 189 calories, 16.6 g fat, 3.1 g protein, 1 g net carbs

Easy Eggs Benedict

These eggs bennys are the easiest thing you've ever made, and oh-so-delicious! Serve them on top of a slice of ham, or your favourite keto-friendly bread for a delectable treat that's ready in minutes!

Serving: 1

Serving Size: whole recipe

Prep Time: 5 minutes

Cook Time: 7 minutes

Ingredients

2 eggs

2 tbsp mayo

1 tbsp olive oil

1 tbsp lemon juice

¼ tsp cayenne

Instructions

Preheat broiler to 500F

To poach the eggs, fill a regular coffee mug with ¼ cup water. Crack in one egg, and cover the cup with a plate or lid. Microwave on high for 50 seconds. Scoop out your perfectly poached egg, and set it aside. Repeat with the second egg.

Meanwhile, whisk together the mayo, olive oil, lemon and cayenne. Place the poached eggs on top of keto-friendly toast, ham, or avocado. Drizzle the hollandaise over the the eggs, and broil for 3-5 minutes. Serve immediately.

Nutrition: 366 calories, 32.8g fat, 11.5g protein, 5 g net carbs

Matcha Smoothie Bowl

This smoothie bowl is exotic and delicious! If you wish, add a bit of spirulina to really amp up the colour and add an extra dose of green power!

Serving: 1

Serving Size: whole recipe

Prep Time: 5 minutes

Cook Time: 0 minutes

Ingredients

2 tsp matcha powder

1 cup coconut milk

1 tbsp chia seeds

1 tbsp coconut flakes

2 tbsp almond slivers

2 tsp spirulina (optional)

Instructions

Mix the coconut milk and matcha together in a bowl. Stir in the spirulina, if using.

 Top with the chia seeds, coconut flakes and almonds. Serve immediately or refrigerate overnight.

Nutrition: 691 calories, 67.9 g fat, 12.9 g protein, 8 g net carbs

Nutty Coffee

A spin on Bulletproof coffee, this flavourful coffee is the perfect thing if you're craving something a bit different

Serving: 1

Serving Size: about 1 ½ cups

Prep Time: 5 minutes

Cook Time: 0 minutes

Ingredients

1 tbsp almond butter

1 tsp cinnamon

1 tsp butter, melted

1 cup freshly brewed coffee

¼ cup almond milk

Instructions

Blend together all ingredients until smooth.

Scotch Eggs

Scotch eggs are traditionally soft-boiled eggs that have been coated in sausage and breading, and deep fried! The perfect Scotch egg is gooey in the center, and crispy on the outside with a thick coating of perfectly seasoned sausage all around.

Serving: 4

Serving Size: 1 egg

Prep Time: 5 minutes

Cook Time: 10 minutes

Ingredients

½ lb ground pork

2 tsp nutmeg

1 tsp dried thyme

Salt and pepper, to taste

4 eggs

1 cup ground pork rinds

6 cups oil, for frying

Instructions

Soft boil the eggs- In a medium sized saucepan with 1 cup of water in the bottom, boil the eggs for 4 minutes. Transfer to an ice bath, and allow to cool. Peel carefully, making sure not to break the eggs.

Mix together the pork, nutmeg, thyme, salt and pepper. Carefully mould the pork mixture around the soft boiled eggs, and roll the mixture in the ground pork rinds.

Pour the oil into a large pot and bring to a temperature of 350f on the stove, using a candy thermometer. Roll the sausage-coated eggs in the pork rinds, and fry for 2-4 minutes, until the eggs begin to float. Remove from heat, drain on a paper towel, and serve immediately.

Nutrition: 442 calories, 46g fat, 25g protein, 0g net carbs

Coconut Smoothie

Coconut and citrus zest come together in this simple smoothie

Serving: 1

Serving Size: Whole Recipe

Prep Time: 5 minutes

Cook Time: 0 minutes

Ingredients

1 cup coconut cream

½ cup crushed ice

1 orange, juice and zest

1 lime, juice and zest

Instructions

In a blender, combine all ingredients until smooth. Serve immediately

Nutrition: 638 calories, 57.4 g fat, 7.2 g protein, 9 g net carbs

Keto Lemon Tea

Classic warm lemon tea is amped up with the addition of coconut oil for a keto morning beverage

Serving: 1

Serving Size: Whole Recipe

Prep Time: 5 minutes

Cook Time: 0 minutes

Ingredients

2 tbsp coconut oil

1 cup boiling water

1 lemon, juice and zest

Instructions

Combine all ingredients, and let sit for 5 minutes. Drink warm.

Nutrition: 251 calories, 27.4 g fat,0.6 g protein, 3 g net carbs

Asparagus Goat Cheese Omelette

This elegant omelette comes together super fast!

Serving: 1

Serving Size: Whole Recipe

Prep Time: 5 minutes

Cook Time: 8 minutes

Ingredients

2 tbsp butter

3 eggs, beaten

¼ cup cream

2 oz goat cheese

2 stalks asparagus, sliced

Instructions

Preheat a pan over medium heat

Beat the eggs and cream with a pinch of salt and pepper

Melt the butter into the pan, then add the asparagus. Pour in the egg mixture

Reduce heat to low, and cook until almost completely cooked through, about 5 minutes.

Flip, and cook the other side for 3 minutes. Top with goat cheese. Serve immediately.

Nutrition: 694 calories, 59.7 g fat, 35 g protein, 4.5 g net carbs

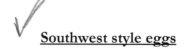

Southwest style eggs

This fun egg recipe combines southwest flavours for a zesty kick to your morning!

Serving: 1

Serving Size: Whole Recipe

Prep Time: 5 minutes

Cook Time: 5 minutes

Ingredients

2 eggs, beaten

¼ cup cream

1 tbsp butter

6 cherry tomatoes, halved

1 tsp cumin

½ tsp chili powder

½ tsp oregano

4 green onions, sliced

¼ cup cheddar cheese, grated

Instructions

Beat the eggs and cream with the seasoning.

Preheat a pan over medium heat, and melt in the butter. Pour in the egg mixture, and cook 2-3 minutes, stirring to scramble. Add in the tomatoes, green onion and cheese, and continue to mix for another 2 minutes.

Serve immediately

Nutrition: 546 calories,35 g fat, 26 g protein, 12 g net carbs

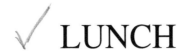

LUNCH

Loaded Avocado Salad

Creamy, salty, and oh-so-satisfying! This avo salad is the perfect midday meal for a busy day!

Serving: 2

Serving Size: 1/2 recipe

Prep Time: 10 minutes

Cook Time: 0 Minutes

Ingredients

2 strips bacon, cooked and chopped into bits

½ avocado, chopped

1 jalapeno, diced (optional)

6 cherry tomatoes, halved

½ cup romaine, chopped

¼ cup blue cheese, crumbled

2 tbsp olive oil

1 tbsp pumpkin seeds

Instructions

Drizzle the oil over the romaine. Toss with the rest of the ingredients. Season with salt and pepper.

Nutrition: 430 calories, 35.5 g fat, 13.2 g protein, 8 g net carb

Keto Lunchables

Just like those compartmentalized lunches you had as a kid, this easy lunch is perfectly portable, easy to put together, and full of all your favourite things! Mix up the contents, but keep the proportions the same in order to maintain your macros.

Serving: 1

Serving Size: Whole recipe

Prep Time: 10 minutes

Cook Time: 0 Minutes

Ingredients

2 oz (about ½ a small breast) cooked chicken breast, sliced

1 hard boiled egg, sliced in half

1 pickle, sliced

4 broccoli florets

4 cauliflower florets

6 grape tomatoes

3 tbsp ranch dressing

*Suggested alternatives- ¼ red pepper, sliced, 4 baby carrots, guacamole, nuts, 2 oz cheese, cooked bacon or ham

Instructions

Place all the individual pieces into their own compartments or individual containers. Nibble and dip as you like.

Nutrition: 590 calories, 37.6 g fat, 28.6 g protein, 6 g net carbs

Salmon and Avocado Nori Rolls

Nori is a delicious, low cal option for wrapping all your favourite foods! Avocado adds a nice amount of good fat, although you can also use a bit of cream cheese for a different flavour profile! Serve alongside some tamari and wasabi for a delectable asian lunch!

Serving: 1

Serving Size: Whole recipe

Prep Time: 10 minutes

Cook Time: 0 Minutes

Ingredients

3 oz cooked salmon

½ avocado, mashed lightly

1 tbsp Sesame seeds

¼ cucumber, cut into sticks (about 4-6 pieces)

1 nori sheet

Instructions

Spread the avocado evenly over the nori sheet.

Flake the salmon over top, and top with the sesame seeds. Lay the cucumber sticks evenly down the side of the sheet. Gently roll the sheet, starting around the cucumber and working up to the other end, to create a maki roll.

Slice into 6 even pieces. Serve with a bit of tamari and wasabi.

Nutrition: 380 calories, 29.6 g fat, 20.6 g protein, 3.5 g net carbs

Smoked salmon Rolls

Smoked salmon and cream cheese are a match made in heaven! These little rolls make an excellent appetizer, but are also great on top of a light green salad for a delicious lunch or light dinner option

Serving: 1

Serving Size: Whole recipe

Prep Time: 10 minutes

Cook Time: 0 Minutes

Ingredients

5 oz smoked salmon

¼ cup cream cheese, softened

Instructions

Spread the cream cheese as evenly as you can over the smoked salmon strips. Roll into pinwheels. Serve immediately, or store in an airtight container in the fridge for up to 1 day.

Nutrition: 368 calories, 26.3g fat, 30 g protein, 1.5 g net carbs

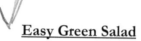

Easy Green Salad

Because of the heart-healthy olive oil, this salad provides an extra boost of fat while also contributing to your daily intake of greens. Perfect for a quick snack, or to add on to any lunch or dinner!

Serving: 1

Serving Size: Whole recipe

Prep Time: 5 minutes

Cook Time: 0 Minutes

Ingredients

1 cup mixed greens (such as baby romaine, baby kale, spinach, or arugula)

Dressing:

2 tbsp olive oil

1 tsp dijon mustard

1 tsp balsamic vinegar

Instructions

Whisk together the oil, dijon and balsamic. Pour the dressing over the greens, and toss well. Season with salt and pepper. Serve immediately

Nutrition: 246 calories, 28.3g fat, 0.4 g protein, 0.1 g net carbs

Tuna Salad Lettuce Wraps

Fast, easy and so delicious! These lettuce wraps have it all!

Serving: 1

Serving Size: Whole recipe

Prep Time: 10 minutes

Cook Time: 0 Minutes

Ingredients

1 can tuna, drained

2 tbsp mayo

1 stalk celery, diced

¼ red pepper, diced

2 tbsp red onion, diced

Salt and pepper, to taste

4 large romaine leaves

Instructions

Mix together all ingredients, except the romaine leaves.

Spoon the mixture into the leaves, and roll into bundles.

Serve immediately, or store in an airtight container in the fridge for up to 1 day.

Nutrition: 466 calories, 24.2 g fat, 48.1 g protein, 7.1 g net carbs

Caprese Salad

This salad is light, quick, and delicious!

Serving: 1

Serving Size: Whole recipe

Prep Time: 3 minutes

Cook Time: 0 Minutes

Ingredients

1 tomato, sliced

2 oz mozzarella, sliced

Handful basil, chopped

3 tbsp olive oil

Handful arugula

1 tbsp balsamic vinegar

Instructions

Arrange the mozzarella, tomato, and basil onto a plate so that each ingredient overlaps each other.

Drizzle with the olive oil and balsamic. Top with the arugula. Serve immediately or keep in an airtight container in the fridge for a day.

Nutrition: 534 calories, 52.2 g fat, 16.6 g protein, 3 g net carbs

 Chicken BLT Salad

A classic sandwich in salad form! Delicious!

Serving: 1

Serving Size: Whole recipe

Prep Time: 5 minutes

Cook Time: 0 Minutes

Ingredients

2 oz cooked chicken, sliced

2 strips bacon, cooked and diced

6 cherry tomatoes, cut in half

1 cup romaine lettuce

¼ cup cheddar cheese, grated

3 tbsp ranch dressing

Instructions

Toss together all ingredients. Serve immediately, or store in an airtight container in the fridge for up to 3 days

Nutrition: 734 calories, 52.5 g fat, 45.1 g protein, 9 g net carbs

Chicken and avocado nori wraps

Nori adds valuable greens and replaces grain-based wraps for this chicken sandwich

Serving: 1

Serving Size: Whole recipe

Prep Time: 5 minutes

Cook Time: 0 Minutes

Ingredients

2 oz cooked chicken, sliced

2 strips bacon, cooked and diced

¼ red pepper, sliced thinly

½ avocado, mashed

1 tbsp hot mustard

2 romaine leaves, chopped

Instructions

Spread the avocado onto the nori sheet. Add in the rest of the ingredients, and roll like a burrito. Serve immediately , or store in the fridge for up to a day.

Nutrition: 657 calories, 50.5 g fat, 33 g protein, 9 g net carbs

DINNER

<u>Lettuce Wrapped Chicken Fajitas</u>

Precooked chicken breasts make this a quick, easy dinner to throw together!

Serving: 1

Serving Size: Whole recipe

Prep Time: 5 minutes

Cook Time: 10 Minutes

Ingredients

4 oz cooked chicken breast

1 tbsp olive oil

¼ red pepper, sliced

¼ red onion, sliced

1 tsp garlic powder

1 tsp cumin

1 tsp chili powder

1 tsp oregano

1 tsp salt

3 large romaine leaves

1 serving Guacamole (*see snack recipes)

3 tbsp salsa

Cilantro, for garnish

Instructions

Preheat a medium pan over medium high heat.

Drizzle in the oil, and add in the peppers, onion, and seasonings. Saute for about 5 minutes.

Add in the chicken breast, and continue to saute for another 5 minutes.

To serve, scoop the chicken and veg into a lettuce leaf, and top with salsa and guac. Garnish with cilantro leaves

Nutrition: 320 calories, 20 g fat, 26.2 g protein, 4 g net carbs

Coconut Lime Noodles and Tofu

Shiritake noodles are low carb and absolutely delicious! Helloooo, keto friendly noodle dishes!

Serving: 2

Serving Size: Half recipe

Prep Time: 5 minutes

Cook Time: 10 Minutes

Ingredients

2 tbsp vegetable oil

1 tsp curry powder

1 tsp cayenne pepper

¼ tsp ground ginger

1 tsp garlic powder

1 lb tofu, diced

1 8oz package shiratake noodles

1/2 can coconut cream

1 tbsp sesame seeds

1 lime, juice and zest

2 tbsp tamari

1 jalapeno, sliced thinly

Handful cilantro, chopped

Instructions

Preheat a medium pan over medium high heat.

Drizzle in the oil, and add in the spices along with the tofu. Toss well for 2 minutes, making sure the tofu is evenly coated on all sides.

Add in the coconut cream and lime juice, and mix well. Add in the noodles straight away, tossing well to combine

Add in the jalapeno, cilantro, tamari, and sesame seeds. Continue to cook for another 5-7 minutes or so, until the sauce has thickened.

Nutrition: 370 calories, 31 g fat, 16 g protein, 4 g net carbs

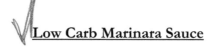

Low Carb Marinara Sauce

Most store bought marinara sauces are loaded with sugar, making them a no-go for the ketogenic diet. Luckily, this tasty marinara sauce is easy to make, super flavourful, and low carb! Use it on veggie noodles, chicken parm, or on anything else you like!

Serving: 4

Serving Size: ¼ cup

Prep Time: 5 minutes

Cook Time: 0 Minutes

Ingredients

1 8oz can crushed tomatoes

2 tbsp dried oregano

1 tbsp dried basil

2 cloves garlic, chopped

½ onion, diced

Salt and pepper, to taste

Handful fresh basil and parsley, chopped

3 tbsp olive oil

Instructions

In a blender or food processor, puree everything together until smooth. Transfer to an airtight container, and store in the refrigerator for up to 5 days. When ready to use, pour desired amount into a saucepan and bring to a boil. Reduce heat to low, and simmer for 5 minutes.

Nutrition: 169 calories, 11.3 g fat, 3.8 g protein, 8 g net carbs

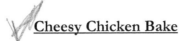

Cheesy Chicken Bake

Using precooked chicken makes this meal come together in a snap! Use homemade marinara sauce to avoid any sugars and additives.

Serving: 2

Serving Size: Half of recipe

Prep Time: 2 minutes

Cook Time: 10 Minutes

Ingredients

2 tbsp olive oil

1 8 oz chicken breast, cooked and sliced

1 tsp dried thyme

1 tsp dried basil

1 tsp dried oregano

1 tsp garlic powder

Salt and pepper, to taste

2 servings marinara sauce (about ½ cup)

¼ cup parmesan cheese

½ cup mozzarella cheese

Instructions

Preheat broiler to 550F.

Toss together the chicken, oil, and seasonings in an oven-proof container. Pour the marinara over top, and cover with cheese.

Broil for 10 minutes, until the cheese is bubbling. Serve warm.

Cream of Broccoli Soup

This soup is a snap to make in a high powered blender! Make a big batch if you like- it'll keep for up to a week in the fridge, and up to 3 months in the freezer!

Serving: 6

Serving Size: 1 cup

Prep Time: 5 minutes

Cook Time: 10 Minutes

Ingredients

½ head broccoli, chopped

½ onion, diced

3 cloves garlic, chopped

½ tsp ground nutmeg

1 tsp dried thyme

3 cups heavy cream

2 cups chicken stock

¼ cup grated parmesan

Instructions

Puree all ingredients together in a high speed blender until smooth.

Transfer the portion you're using immediately to a saucepan big enough to hold it comfortably. Keep the rest in an airtight container in the fridge for up to 14 days, or freeze in individual portions for up to 3 months.

Cook over medium-high heat for 10 minutes, until heated through.

Nutrition: 232 calories, 22.8 g fat, 2.9 g protein, 3 g net carbs

Avocado BLT

Avo buns are all the rage, and this easy sandwich is satisfying and fun to eat!

Serving: 1

Serving Size: whole recipe

Prep Time: 5 minutes

Cook Time: 0 Minutes

Ingredients

1 avocado. Sliced in half

2 strips bacon, cooked

1 slice tomato

1 ring red onion

1 leaf romaine lettuce

½ tbsp mayo

½ tbsp dijon mustard

½ tsp sesame seeds

Instructions

Using the avocado as your "bun", spread on the mayo and mustard, and layer in the bacon, tomato, onion, and lettuce.

Close the sandwich, and sprinkle sesame seeds on top of the avocado bun for a fun look! Slice in half, and serve immediately.

Nutrition: 540 calories, 46.1 g fat, 18.3 g protein, 5.6 g net carbs

Salmon Putanesca

Who doesn't love flavourful tomatoes, olives and herbs over a good quality piece of fish? Purchase wild, sustainably caught salmon.

Serving: 2

Serving Size: 1 piece fish

Prep Time: 5 minutes

Cook Time: 15 Minutes

Ingredients

2 3 oz fillets salmon

8 cherry tomatoes, halved

2 oz anchovies, finely chopped

6 kalamata olives, pitted and chopped

1 tbsp olive oil

Handful fresh basil and parsley

Salt and pepper, to taste

Instructions

Preheat oven to 375F

Preheat a small pan over medium heat, Drizzle in the olive oil and add in the anchovies, tomatoes, olives, and herbs. Saute for about 3 minutes.

Lay the fish onto a baking sheet lined with parchment, and season with salt and pepper. Spoon the tomato mixture evenly over both pieces of fish, and bake for 10-12 minutes, until the fish is cooked through. Serve warm, and keep any leftovers in a tightly sealed container in the fridge for up to 2 days.

Nutrition: 600 calories, 30.3 g fat, 72.4 g protein, 8 g net carbs

Ham and Swiss Cheese Crustless Quiche

What's the difference between a frittata and a crustless quiche? Not much, actually! But you can definitely impress your friends and family with this fancy sounding name, and make an awesome one pan meal while you're at it!

Serving: 2

Serving Size: Half recipe

Prep Time: 5 minutes

Cook Time: 11 Minutes

Ingredients

1 tbsp butter

4 oz ham, cubed

4 oz swiss cheese, grated

4 eggs, beaten

1 tbsp mayo

¼ cup heavy cream

¼ cup spinach

Salt and pepper, to taste

Instructions

Preheat oven to 375F

Preheat a medium sized, oven safe pan over medium heat on the stovetop. Melt in the butter, and saute the spinach for 1 minute. Remove from heat.

Beat together the eggs, mayo, cream, salt and pepper. Pour the mixture over the spinach, and add in the rest of the ingredients.

Transfer the pan to the oven, and bake for 10-12 minutes until cooked through.

Nutrition: 566 calories, 43.2 g fat, 36.3g protein, 5.6 g net carbs

 <u>**Chicken a la King**</u>

Have you ever had this vintage dish? It's creamy and comforting, and the perfect way to end your day! Cooked chicken breasts make this dish come together super fast! Eat on its own, or serve alongside a green salad if you like

Serving: 1

Serving Size: Whole recipe

Prep Time: 5 minutes

Cook Time: 15 Minutes

Ingredients

1 tbsp butter

4 oz cooked chicken breast, sliced

3 oz mushrooms, sliced

1 clove garlic, minced

¼ onion, diced

½ carrot, diced

½ cup heavy cream

¼ red pepper, diced

Instructions

Preheat a medium sized pan over medium high heat. Melt in the butter, and saute the mushrooms, carrot, garlic and onion with a pinch of pepper. Add in the cream, and stir well.

Add in the chicken and red pepper, stirring well for 3-5 minutes.

Reduce heat to medium low, and simmer another 10 minutes or so, until the sauce has thickened slightly and a stew-like consistency is achieved. Serve warm.

Nutrition: 494 calories, 36.9 g fat, 29.1 g protein, 4.3 g net carbs

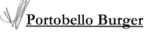 **Portobello Burger**

This yummy burger uses two portobello mushrooms as the bun!

Serving: 1

Serving Size: Whole recipe

Prep Time: 5 minutes

Cook Time: 15 Minutes

Ingredients

¼ lb ground beef

1 egg

1 tsp garlic powder

Salt and pepper to taste

1 oz mozzarella cheese, grated

1 tomato slice

1 ring red onion

Handful arugula or 1 romaine leaf

2 portobello caps

1 tbsp oil

Instructions

Preheat oven to 375f

Brush the mushrooms with oil, and season with salt and pepper.

Mix together the beef, egg, garlic, salt and pepper. Form into a patty.

Lay the patty alongside the mushroom caps on a baking sheet lined with parchment. Bake 15 minutes.

Lay the cooked patty on top of one of the mushroom caps. Top with the cheese, tomato, onion and greens. Close the burger with the remaining cap. Serve warm.

Nutrition: 485 calories, 30 g fat, 48.6 g protein, 2 g net carbs

Shrimp Stir Fry

This stir fry uses guilt-free shiratake noodles, along with delicious shrimp and a variety of keto friendly veg for a really yummy dinner or lunch option!

Serving: 2

Serving Size: Half recipe

Prep Time: 5 minutes

Cook Time: 10 Minutes

Ingredients

2 tbsp sesame oil

1 orange, juice and zest

2 tbsp tamari

1 tbsp ginger

1 tbsp sesame seeds

2 cloves garlic, minced

3 red chilies, finely sliced

3 tbsp coconut oil

¼ onion, sliced finely

1 celery stalk, finely sliced

6 oz oyster mushrooms, torn

½ red pepper, sliced

12 jumbo shrimp, peeled and deveined

1 8oz package shiratake noodles

Instructions

Rinse the noodles well in a colander, and pat dry.

Preheat a wok or medium sized pan over medium high heat. Melt in the coconut oil, and add in the onion, celery, mushrooms and peppers. Saute for 2 minutes, until softened slightly. Add in the shrimp, and continue to saute for another 3 minutes.

Drizzle in the sesame oil, and add in the garlic, ginger, tamari and orange. Toss well for 2 minutes.

Add the shiratake noodles, and toss well. Continue cooking for another 5 minutes until the sauce has thickened slightly and coats the noodles. Serve warm, and store any leftovers in an airtight container for up to 3 days.

Nutrition: 600 calories, 56 g fat, 30.6 g protein, 7 g net carbs

Middle Eastern Style Stuffed Tomatoes

Ground beef, pine nuts, tomatoes and a drizzle of decadent tahini! What else could you want in a dinner?

Serving: 2

Serving Size: 1 tomato

Prep Time: 5 minutes

Cook Time: 15 Minutes

Ingredients

2 tbsp olive oil

¼ lb ground beef

¼ onion, diced

1 tsp garlic powder

1 tsp cumin

1 tsp coriander powder

1 tsp turmeric

1 tsp chili powder

2 tbsp pine nuts

Handful parsley, chopped

2 tomatoes, cut in half through the center (to make 4 shells)

¼ cup tahini (found in snack recipes)

Instructions

Preheat the oven to 450F.

Preheat a medium pan over medium high heat. Drizzle in the oil, and add the onion and seasonings. Saute for 1 minute, then add in the beef. Continue cooking for 5-7 minutes, until the beef is cooked through.

Lay the tomatoes onto a baking sheet, and spoon in the beef. Bake for 5 minutes.

To serve, drizzle with tahini and top with parsley.

Nutrition: 400 calories, 33 g fat, 22.9 g protein, 5 g net carbs

Ma Po Tofu

This spicy Szechuan dish incorporates bright flavours and tofu and ground beef. Eat on its own, or serve on top of a bed or shiratake noodles or cauliflower rice

Serving: 2

Serving Size: Half Recipe

Prep Time: 5 minutes

Cook Time: 15 Minutes

Ingredients

1 lb silken tofu

100 g ground beef

1 tbsp sesame oil

3 red chilies, finely chopped

2 tbsp tamari

1 cup beef stock

2 tbsp coconut oil

3 green onions, finely sliced

1 tsp ginger

2 cloves garlic, minced

¼ cup broccoli florets, steamed

Instructions

Mix together the beef and sesame oil with a pinch of salt, and set aside.

Dice the tofu into cubes, and submerge in boiling water with a pinch of salt. Set aside.

Preheat a wok over medium high heat. Melt in the coconut oil, then fry the beef for about 3 minutes. Spoon the beef onto a plate and set aside.

Drizzle in a bit more sesame oil, and add the green onion, ginger, garlic and chilies. Saute for 2 minutes until fragrant.

Add the beef stock and tofu, and bring to a boil. Add the beef back in, and cook for another 8 minutes, stirring well until the liquid has evaporated slightly. Add the tamari. Taste, and adjust seasoning as needed.

Serve with broccoli florets, and some cauliflower rice if you like.

Nutrition: 449 calories, 30.1 g fat, 35.1 g protein, 6 g net carbs

Bacon Butter Cod

This cod is deliciously decadent, and very easy to prepare! Serve with an easy green salad, or with a serving of parmesan crusted cauliflower for a complete meal.

Serving: 2

Serving Size: Half Recipe

Prep Time: >1 minute

Cook Time: 20 Minutes

Ingredients

2 4 oz fillets cod

4 strips bacon, diced

2 tbsp butter

1 tsp dried thyme

Salt and pepper to taste

Instructions

Preheat oven to 350F

Pat the cod dry, and season with salt and pepper. Bake for 15-20 minutes.

Meanwhile, preheat a small pan over medium heat. Cook the bacon and butter together, stirring constantly for about 3 minutes until the bacon is fully cooked. Add in the thyme, and continue to cook for another minute or so, being careful not to burn the bacon or the butter.

Once the fish has cooked, spoon the butter-bacon mixture over top. Serve immediately.

Nutrition: 323 calories, 27.6 g fat, 17.5 g protein, 0.7 g net carbs

 ## Parmesan Roasted Cauliflower

This yummy side dish is the perfect addition to any meal, but also makes a great lunch or snack on its own. Swap out the cauliflower for broccoli if you're looking to incorporate a bit more green into your diet.

Serving: 2

Serving Size: Half Recipe

Prep Time: 5 minutes

Cook Time: 15 Minutes

Ingredients

½ head cauliflower, cut into florets

¼ cup olive oil

1 tsp salt

1 tsp garlic powder

½ cup parmesan, grated

Instructions

Preheat oven to 400F

Toss together all ingredients. Lay onto a baking sheet lined with parchment, and bake for 15 minutes. Serve warm, or keep in an airtight container in the fridge for up to a week.

Nutrition: 260 calories, 26.8 g fat, 35.1 g protein, 6 g net carbs

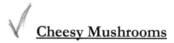 <u>**Cheesy Mushrooms**</u>

These mushrooms are easy, quick and delicious!

Serving: 2

Serving Size: Half Recipe

Prep Time: 5 minutes

Cook Time: 15 Minutes

Ingredients

2 portobello mushroom caps

¼ cup mozzarella cheese, shredded

1 tbsp olive oil

1 cup spinach

1 tbsp butter, room temp

Instructions

Preheat oven to 400F

Brush the mushrooms with the oil, and season with a bit of salt and pepper.

Mix together the butter and spinach, and press the mixture into the center of the mushroom caps.

Top with the cheese, and bake for 15 minutes. Serve warm.

Nutrition: 124 calories, 13.5 g fat, 1.5 g protein, 0.2 g net carbs

Bacon-tomato-cheddar soup

This soup is so rich and satisfying, you'll want to have it every night!

Serving: 4

Serving Size: 1 cup

Prep Time: 5 minutes

Cook Time: 15 Minutes

Ingredients

¼ onion, diced

1 can crushed tomatoes

1 tbsp dried thyme

1 cup chicken stock

1 cup cream

1 clove garlic

½ cup cheddar cheese, grated

2 tbsp butter

4 strips bacon, diced

Instructions

In a blender, puree together the tomato, garlic, chicken stock, onion and thyme.

In a large saucepan over medium heat, melt the butter and fry the bacon for 1 minute. Add the tomato mixture, and bring to a boil.

Reduce the heat to low, and simmer for 10 minutes. Add the cream, and simmer for another 2-3 minutes. Stir in the cheese. Serve immediately.

Nutrition: 270 calories, 21.9 g fat, 12.2 g protein, 1 g net carbs

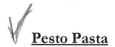

Pesto Pasta

A super easy pesto on top of zucchini noodles is the perfect quick dinner for a busy weeknight!

Serving: 2

Serving Size: Half of recipe

Prep Time: 5 minutes

Cook Time: 10 Minutes

Ingredients

3 cups basil

2 cloves garlic

¼ cup pine nuts

½ cup parmesan, grated

¼ cup olive oil

4 zucchinis, spiralized

Instructions

In a blender, puree together the basil, garlic, pine nuts, parm and oil.

Preheat a large pan over medium heat. Add in the pesto and zucchini noodles, and toss well to combine. Cook for about 10 minutes until cooked through. Serve immediately or keep leftovers in a container in the fridge for up to 3 days.

Nutrition: 646 calories, 53.8 g fat, 32.4g protein, 10 g net carbs

 ### Cheesy Meatballs

This dish is so fast to make, and really yummy! Serve it with Marinara for a quick, satisfying meal. Make a big batch in advance, and freeze them for a quick, satisfying meal any time!

Serving: 2

Serving Size: 4 meatballs

Prep Time: 5 minutes

Cook Time: 15 Minutes

Ingredients

¼ lb ground beef

¼ lb ground pork

1 tbsp garlic powder

1 tbsp dried oregano

1 tbsp dried thyme

1 egg, beaten

½ cup mozzarella, shredded

2 servings Low Carb Marinara Sauce

Instructions

Preheat oven to 375F

Mix together all ingredients except the marinara. Form into 8 balls, and lay on a baking sheet lined with parchment.

Bake for 10-12 minutes

Meanwhile, warm the sauce in a large pan over medium high heat

Once the meatballs have cooked, transfer to the pan with the sauce and cook together for 3-5 minutes

Nutrition: 331 calories, 20.6 g fat, 40.1 g protein, 10 g net carbs

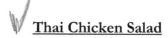

Thai Chicken Salad

This salad comes together quickly, and can be made up to five days in advance!

Serving: 2

Serving Size: Half recipe

Prep Time: 10 minutes

Cook Time: 0 Minutes

Ingredients

6 oz cooked chicken, shredded

1 carrot, grated

½ cucumber, grated or spiralized

1 jalapeno, finely sliced

3 green onions, finely sliced

2 tbsp mayo

1 tbsp curry powder

2 tbsp coconut cream

1 tsp garlic powder

1 tsp ginger

½ cup bean sprouts

1 tsp sesame oil

Instructions

Whisk together the curry powder, garlic, ginger, mayo and coconut cream. Add in all the other ingredients, and toss well to combine. Store in an airtight container for up to 5 days.

Nutrition: 303 calories, 14.2 g fat, 28.9 g protein, 9.1 g net carbs

Southwest Chicken Avocado Salad

This fun salad is so yummy and healthy! You'll love it!

Serving: 1

Serving Size: whole recipe

Prep Time: 5 minutes

Cook Time: 0 Minutes

Ingredients

4 oz cooked chicken breast, sliced

¼ cup cheddar cheese, grated

1 avocado, diced

¼ red pepper, diced

6 cherry tomatoes, halved

1 jalapeno, diced

1 lime, juice and zest

1 tsp garlic powder

1 tsp cayenne

Instructions

Mix together all ingredients, tossing well to combine. Serve immediately, or keep in the fridge for up to 6 hours.

Nutrition: 800 calories 53.1 g fat, 41.9 g protein, 5 g net carbs

Baked Cod with Lemony Asparagus

A one pan meal that is easy, tasty and healthy!

Serving: 2

Serving Size:half recipe

Prep Time: >1 minutes

Cook Time: 20 Minutes

Ingredients

2 4 oz fillets cod

1 tsp thyme

8 stalks asparagus, trimmed

3 tbsp olive oil

Salt and pepper, to taste

1 lemon, juice and zest, PLUS

1 lemon, cut into wheels

Instructions

Preheat oven to 350F

Sprinkle the thyme and some salt and pepper over the fish

Lay the lemon wheels down on a baking sheet lined with parchment. Lay the fish on top of the lemon wheels.

Toss the asparagus in the oil, salt and pepper and lemon zest and juice. Lay it beside the fish on the baking sheet.

Bake 20 minutes. Serve immediately, and refrigerate any leftovers for 1 day.

Nutrition: 554 calories 26 g fat, 81 g protein, 1.3 g net carbs

Asparagus, smoked salmon and goat cheese salad

The perfect healthy salad to end your day

Serving: 1

Serving Size: whole recipe

Prep Time: 10 minutes

Cook Time: 0 Minutes

Ingredients

6 oz smoked salmon

1 oz goat cheese

6 stalks asparagus, sliced

Handful arugula

1 lemon, juice and zest

1 tbsp olive oil

Instructions

Mix the lemon juice, zest and olive oil together

Add in the arugula, and toss well to combine

Mix in the goat cheese, asparagus and salmon.

Serve immediately

Nutrition: 466 calories 31.6 g fat, 41.9 g protein, 2.3 g net carbs

SNACKS

<u>Veggie Sticks and Guacamole</u>

This creamy guac is loaded with fat and nutrients! Double up on the recipe and keep it in an airtight container in the fridge for up to 2 days, so that you can have it on-hand for whenever a craving strikes! Veggie sticks add a boost of nutrition, and are perfect for dipping.

Serving: 1

Serving Size: Whole Recipe

Prep Time: 10 minutes

Cook Time: 0 Minutes

Ingredients

½ avocado

1 lime, zest and juice

3 tbsp cilantro, chopped

½ jalapeno, diced

1 clove garlic, minced

Veggies:

¼ red pepper, cut into strips

1 stalk celery, cut into sticks

2 baby carrots, cut in half

Instructions

Preheat oven to 185C/375F. Wash and dry the kale fully, and chop it into large pieces. Toss it with the oil, and the rest of the ingredients.

Lay the dressed kale onto a baking sheet lined with parchment paper. Bake for 30 minutes, until crispy and fragrant.

Allow to cool fully. Portion the kale chips into two airtight containers, and store up to a week at room temperature.

Nutrition: 240 calories, 20.1 g fat, 4 g protein, 3.6 g net carbs

Almond Coconut Fat Bombs

Fat bombs are easy and fun to make! Although they do need time to set in the freezer, they take no time at all to whip up. These fat bombs contain coconut, almonds and chocolate.

Serving: 12

Serving Size: 1 fat bomb

Prep Time: >5 minutes

Cook Time: 1 Minute

Ingredients

¼ cup almond butter

¼ cup coconut oil

2 tbsp erythritol

¼ cup unsweetened coconut flakes

2 tbsp cocoa powder

Instructions

Mix together the coconut oil and almond butter in a microwave safe bowl, and microwave on high for 1 minute.

Stir in the rest of the ingredients.

Pour into 12 individual cupcake papers, and freeze for at least 10 minutes. Allow the fat bomb to come to room temperature before eating. Store fat bombs in a ziplock bag or airtight container in the freezer for up to 6 months.

Nutrition: 200 calories, 20 g fat, 3 g protein, 2 g net carbs

Tahini with veggie sticks

Tahini is a delicious middle eastern sauce made with sesame paste (also called tahini), garlic, lemon and herbs. Use it on top of anything that needs a boost of flavour and fat, or as a dip for veggies for a satisfying snack

Serving: 4

Serving Size: 3 tbsp

Prep Time: 10 minutes

Cook Time: 0 Minutes

Ingredients

3 tbsp tahini paste

1 lemon, juice and zest

1 clove garlic

Handful parsley, chopped

Salt, to taste

½ cup water

Veggies:

¼ red pepper, cut into strips

1 stalk celery, cut into sticks

2 baby carrots, cut in half

Instructions

In a blender or food processor, combine all ingredients until smooth.

Transfer to an airtight container and keep in the fridge for up to 7 days. Serve with your favourite veggies for a guilt free, full fat snack!

Nutrition: 89 calories, 8 g fat, 2.6 g protein, 1 g net carbs

Guacamole Deviled Eggs

Serving: 6

Serving Size: 2 Pieces

Prep Time: 10 minutes

Cook Time: 0 Minutes

Ingredients

6 Eggs, hardboiled

1 Avocado, mashed

1 Tbsp lime juice

1 jalapeno, diced

Salt and pepper to taste

Instructions

Peel the eggs, and slice in half. Remove the yolks, and transfer to a bowl with the rest of the ingredients. Set the whites aside for a moment.

Mash together the yolks, avocado, jalapeno and lime juice with the salt and pepper. If you like, add a pinch of cayenne.

Spoon the filling into the eggs. Eat immediately, or keep in an airtight container in the fridge for up to a week.

Nutrition: 195 calories, 17g fat, 7g protein, 3g net carbs

Caprese rolls with prosciutto

These simple rolls are the perfect snack to make on a busy evening! Because of the classic combination of salty, creamy and herby, they also make a great topping for a simple salad.

Serving: 1

Serving Size: 4 Pieces

Prep Time: 10 minutes

Cook Time: 0 Minutes

Ingredients

50 g sliced prosciutto

25 g mozzarella, sliced

4 large basil leaves

1 small tomato, sliced

1 tsp balsamic vinegar

Instructions

Lay the prosciutto out onto a plate or cutting board.

Layer the mozzarella over top, followed by the basil. Roll the prosciutto to form a wheel, so the cheese and basil are inside the meat.

Slice in half, and lay each piece on top of a slice of tomato.

Drizzle with balsamic. Serve immediately, or refrigerate up to 48 hours.

Nutrition: 95 calories, 4g fat, 12.5g protein, 1 g net carbs

 Coconut Matcha Fat Bombs

Matcha powder is rich in antioxidants, and tastes fantastic! You'll love this asian inspired fat bomb!

Serving: 12

Serving Size: 1 fat bomb

Prep Time: 15 minutes

Cook Time: 0 minutes

Ingredients

½ cup coconut oil

½ cup coconut cream

1 tsp matcha powder

1 tbsp powdered stevia

¼ tsp salt

½ tsp vanilla extract

For the topping:

2 tbsp coconut flakes

1 tbsp matcha powder

Instructions

In a bowl, combine the coconut flakes and 1 teaspoon of matcha powder, and set aside.

In another bowl, beat together the rest of the ingredients using a hand mixer, or combine in a standing mixer using the whisk attachment until light and fluffy.

Spoon out 12 equal sized scoops onto a baking sheet lined with parchment. Roll each scoop into a ball, and drop into the coconut-matcha topping. Roll around until completely covered.

Freeze for at least 20 minutes, and keep in the freezer for up to 6 months.

Lt the fat bomb sit at room temperature for 15 minutes before eating.

Nutrition: 100 calories, 11.5 g fat, 0.2 g protein, 2g net carbs

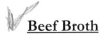

Beef Broth

Beef broth is easy to make, and really good for you! The addition of coconut oil adds a ton of flavour, while also increasing your fat levels

Serving: 1

Serving Size: 1 cup

Prep Time: 0 minutes

Cook Time: 15 minutes

Ingredients

1 cup beef stock

Salt and pepper to taste

1 tsp dried thyme (optional)

2 tbsp coconut oil

Instructions

In a medium sized pot, warm all ingredients over medium high heat. Bring to a boil, and then reduce to low and simmer for 10-12 minutes.

Nutrition: 273 calories, 28.6 g fat, 4.9 g protein, 0.9 g net carbs

Weekly Shopping List

*Note- It can be more economical to purchase meat items in bulk. Portioning out your meat items and freezing them will save time and money later.

*Most of the recipes in this meal plan call for cooked chicken breast and cooked bacon. This has been done as a way to save you time during the week. Plan a prep day each week, read over your meal plan and recipes, and cook your proteins as needed in advance.

For cooked bacon:

Preheat oven to 350F. Lay 1 lb bacon onto a baking sheet lined with parchment. Bake 20-25 minutes, until cooked through. Allow to cool, and portion as needed for the week.

For cooked chicken:

Preheat oven to 350F. Pat the chicken breast dry, and season as you like (recommended per breast- 1 tsp dried thyme, 1 tsp salt, 1 tsp pepper). Pour ¼ cup water into the bottom of a baking sheet, cover with parchment, and lay down the chicken breasts (the steam from the water helps the chicken stay moist). Bake 20-25 minutes until cooked through. Allow to cool, and portion as needed for the week.

Pantry Staples For the Month:

Spirulina- 1 oz

Coconut Milk- 10 cans

Pickles- 1 jar

Kalamata Olives- 8 oz

Almond Butter- 1 jar (about 8 oz)

Stevia (*may sub for Erythritol) - 1 package about 2.5 oz

Sesame Seeds - 4 oz

Almonds - 8 oz

Pecans- 6 oz

Shredded Unsweetened Coconut - 1 lb

Walnuts - 1 lb

Pumpkin Seeds - 1 lb

Flax Seeds - 1 lb
Coconut oil- 1 oz

Canned tomatoes- 4x 8 oz cans
Olive oil mayonnaise or avocado oil mayonnaise - 1 container, about 1 L

Tahini Paste - 1 container, about 1 lb

Italian Herbs- 1 package, about 300g

Dried Thyme- 1 package, about 300g

Cayenne Powder- 1 package, about 300g

Curry Powder- 1 package, about 300g

Cumin- 1 package, about 300g

Ground Ginger- 1 package, about 300g

Sugar Free Sriracha Sauce- 1 bottle

Gluten Free Tamari - 1 bottle

Coffee- 1 lb

Matcha Powder- 300 g

Salt

Pepper

Tortillas- 36 (keep wrapped and sealed until ready to use)

Nori sheets- 1 package

Almond Milk- 4 L

Beef Stock- either 3L prepared, or bouillon cubes

Chicken Stock- either 3L prepared, or bouillon cubes

Shiratake Noodles- 6 packages (keep refrigerated)

Week 1 Shopping List

Seafood, Meat and Eggs:

Eggs- 1 dozen

Salmon- 12 oz (4x 3 oz fillets)

Chicken breast, boneless skinless- 6]oz

Smoked Salmon- 1 lb

Bacon- 1 lb

Tofu- 1 lb

Ham- 1 package (about 6 oz)

Prosciutto- 6 oz

Dairy Products:

Cheddar cheese- 1 lb

Butter- 1 lb

Heavy Cream- 1 L

Mozzarella- 3 oz

Parmesan Cheese- 4 oz

Produce:

6 Avocados

2 Limes

2 Lemons

1 Head of Romaine

1 Package Fresh Spinach

1 Package Fresh Basil

2 peppers

6 jalapenos

1 pint cherry tomatoes

1 cucumber

1 package carrots

1 head broccoli

1 package (8oz) bean sprouts

2 roma tomatoes

1 lb carrots

Celery- 1 head

Week 2 Shopping List

Meat and Eggs:

Salmon- 8oz

Cod- 8 oz

Chicken Breast- 16 oz

Ground beef- 1 lb

Tuna, canned- 1

Bacon- 1 lb

Eggs- 1 dozen

Dairy Products:

None

Produce:

4 Portobello Mushrooms

2 roma tomatoes

1 Pint Cherry Tomatoes

3 lemons

6 Avocados

1 lb Spinach

1 head Romaine Lettuce

1 lb bean sprouts

10 stalks asparagus

1 orange

1 lime

1 red onion

Week 3 Shopping List

Meat and Eggs:

Cod- 6 oz

Shrimp- 1 lb

Ground Pork- 12 oz

Ham- 4 oz

Bacon- 1 lb

Eggs- 1 dozen

Salmon- 8 oz

Chicken breasts- 24 oz

Ground Beef - 8 oz

Dairy Products:

Butter- 1 lb

goat cheese - 8 oz

Cheddar Cheese- 1 lb

Produce:

1 orange

7 Avocados

1 Lime

½ lb Spinach

1 Package Fresh Basil

1 Bunch Cilantro

1 bunch green onions

1 Head of Broccoli

1 Head of Cauliflower

Portobello mushrooms x4

1 head celery

1 bunch carrots

1 tomato

1 package cherry tomatoes

1 red onion

Week 4 Shopping List

Meat and Eggs:

Chicken Breast-1 lb

Proscuitto- 8 oz

Cod- 6 oz

Bacon 1 lb

Eggs- 1 dozen

Shrimp-8 oz

Ham- 8 oz

Salmon- 6 oz

Smoked Salmon- 1 lb

Dairy Products:

Goat Cheese- 8 oz

Heavy Cream- 8 oz

Butter 1 lb

Produce:

1 bunch Asparagus

6 Avocados

1 package spinach

3 Packages Fresh Basil

1 Head Cauliflower

1 Carrot

1 Red Bell Pepper

1 Cucumber

1 Tomato

1 pint cherry tomatoes

4 Onions

2 lemons

1 lime

1 orange

CHAPTER 6
Questions You Will Ask

In this chapter, we will cover some commonly asked questions that pertain to the keto diet. This book is about helping you better understand your keto journey and getting the right information. Hopefully, your most burning questions will be answered in this chapter.

Is it OK to be in ketosis on a long-term basis?

In short, yes! As we talked about in other chapters, we are all born in a state of ketosis and it is not harmful at all. Naturally, as you stay true to the keto diet, your body will use up all its ketone stores and will begin to burn fat for fuel. This is called "fat adaptation". This is the ultimate goal of the kept diet and means that your body is now soley using fat as a source of fuel. You may even notice that your ketone monitors aren't registering ketones, anymore. Don't freak out! Over time, this is what is supposed to happen.

Is it OK to cycle in and out of ketosis?

Depending on your lifestyle, cycling in and out of ketosis is fine, especially if you are a major athlete or body builder. These folks are the only folks who actually need some glycogen before working out or competing. The quick release of sugar goes directly to their muscles and helps them to recover.

Some people find that carb-cycling helps them keep their body from becoming used to the keto diet and helps with weight loss stalls. You'll have to play around with what works best for you.

Can I be a vegetarian and eat a keto diet?

Honestly? Being a vegetarian or a vegan is pretty hard to accomplish while on a ketogenic diet. Many staple foods, like butter, cheese, and meat, are part of the diet. Since the keto diet requires you to cut out starching vegetables and almost all fruits, a vegetarian would be left with barely any food choices at the end of the day. I don't recommend vegetarians follow a keto diet for nutritional purposes.

How long before I see improved health and weight loss?

There is no cookie cutter answer for this question. Everyone is different, and our bodies adapt to new things at their own paces. You must factor in how much weight you need to lose and the severity of the health problems you are having. Some folks see results very quickly while others have to wait a little while as their body adjusts to the new way of eating.

Will I experience kidney stones on the keto WOE?

If you have suffered from kidney stones in the past the likelihood of them returning is probable. However, removing sugar from your diet and watching your mineral and protein intake can help decrease this risk. People who have never had kidney stones rarely develop them from the keto diet.

Why am I losing muscle on keto?

There will always be a degree of muscle loss on any weight loss diet. However, you can minimize this effect by eating adequate amounts of protein. Exercising most days of the week will also be beneficial to keeping your muscle alive and well.

TIPS AND STRATEGIES TO SUSTAINING YOUR KETO LIFESTYLE

Now that you are on the road to better health and weight loss through the ketogenic diet it is time to talk about how to sustain your newfound lifestyle.

Here are a few tips on how you can be successful and sustain all the progress you've made through keto:

1. Sometimes, ketogenic eating can be expensive. Just know that you don't need all the fancy products that you see being touted on keto blogs. So, you can't afford almond meal and MCT oil? No worries! Purchase the keto-friendly foods that you can afford. You can also purchase many keto foods in bulk and freeze, vacuum seal, or can them as this will save you a lot of money.
2. Always keep keto-safe foods within reach. When you are hungry and/or craving you want to have chopped up veggies, sliced cheese, or nuts at your disposal. If you don't have keto-foods ready to go you are more susceptible to reaching for a candy bar.
3. Meal prepping is essential to ketogenic success. Choose one day out of the week and make your meal plans and prep your food for the next 7 days. Sure, it may be labor intensive and time-consuming at first but you'll relish the ease of having your meals already prepped and ready over the course of the next week.
4. Would your family be open to keto? It is so much easier to prepare one type of food instead of two. See if you can't get them onboard the keto train. In fact, keto food tastes so good, my family doesn't even know when they are eating it. I have always made keto suppers for the family and myself. Unlike low-calorie diets, high-fat food is delicious. It's hard to believe that it is actually "diet food".
5. You do not need to exercise in order to be successful on the keto diet. However, it does help things move along a little quicker and it is good for you. Start out small with doing simple walking a few days a week. Gradually, you can move towards a more intense workout routine if you so desire.
6. Lastly, get yourself more keto recipe and research books. You want to keep your meals rotating so you don't get bored. Boredom leads to failure. Explore keto blogs, YouTube channels, and Facebook pages. Look up Dr. Eric Berg and Dr. Jason Fung who are known in the keto community for their expertise on the diet.

CONCLUSION

What Keto Has Meant for Me

Life changer. That is what keto has meant for me. I was tired of feeling sluggish, gaining weight, and having constant bloat around my middle. It hurt me every time I'd wander into a department store and try on clothes only to be disappointed by what I saw staring back at me in the dressing room mirror. Many times, I'd leave the clothes in a crumpled-up ball on the floor and walk out.
Before keto, I had no idea what metabolic syndrome was and that I was being affected by it. Nixing sugar from my diet totally helped repair this ailment. Today, I feel stronger, lighter, and far more fit than I ever have before.

I can run around the yard with my kids, go on hikes, and wake up rested all due to my ketogenic lifestyle. The days of being overweight, exhausted, and feeling frumpy are well behind me.

They can be for you, too.

This book is intended to help folks who are just starting out on the ketogenic diet. It is a guide to helping them meet their health and weight loss goals. It by no means replaces the expertise of your health care professional.

If you are already on a ketogenic diet this book will help you get more out of the lifestyle. Basically, it will help you cross over into more information and a better understanding of why you are choosing the keto WOE.

If you are a fast-paced person with a busy lifestyle, this book is for you as it provides you with a comprehensive quick recipe meal plan. More traditional? No problem. I have a meal plan for you, too.

Lastly, and most importantly, this book has been designed to help people sustain their keto lifestyle for the long haul. It is so important that you remember how you got sick and overweight in the first place and what keto did to change all of that.

Resources

1. https://www.ncbi.nlm.nih.gov/pubmed/17332207
2. https://www.ncbi.nlm.nih.gov/pmc/articles/PMC2633336/
3. https://www.ncbi.nlm.nih.gov/pubmed/11581442
4. https://www.ncbi.nlm.nih.gov/pmc/articles/PMC1819381/
5. https://www.ncbi.nlm.nih.gov/pmc/articles/PMC2367001/
6. https://www.ncbi.nlm.nih.gov/pubmed/14525681
7. https://www.ncbi.nlm.nih.gov/pubmed/6865776
8. https://www.ncbi.nlm.nih.gov/pubmed/14769489
9. https://www.ncbi.nlm.nih.gov/pubmed/14527626
10. https://www.ncbi.nlm.nih.gov/pmc/articles/PMC2633336/
11. https://www.ncbi.nlm.nih.gov/pmc/articles/PMC5329646/
12. https://www.ncbi.nlm.nih.gov/pmc/articles/PMC3826507/
13. https://www.journals.elsevier.com/diabetes-and-metabolic-syndrome-clinical-research-and-reviews
14. https://www.nap.edu/read/10490/chapter/8#275
15. https://www.healthline.com/nutrition/low-carb-ketogenic-diet-brain#section3
16. https://www.ncbi.nlm.nih.gov/pubmed/19332337
17. https://www.ncbi.nlm.nih.gov/pmc/articles/PMC3157418/
18. https://www.ncbi.nlm.nih.gov/pmc/articles/PMC4124736/
19. https://www.ruled.me/the-ketogenic-diet-and-cholesterol/
20. https://www.ruled.me/can-low-carb-diet-lower-blood-pressure/
21. https://www.ruled.me/keto-best-fatty-liver-diet/
22. https://www.ruled.me/3-reasons-keto-better-for-brain/
23. https://www.healthline.com/health/ketosis-vs-ketoacidosis#diagnosis
24. https://ketogasm.com/what-are-macros/
25. https://www.ncbi.nlm.nih.gov/pmc/articles/PMC3257631/

CPSIA information can be obtained
at www.ICGtesting.com
Printed in the USA
LVHW102202290119
605742LV00030B/468/P